ARTHRITIS

A CLEVELAND CLINIC GUIDE

John D. Clough, M.D.

ARTHRITIS: A CLEVELAND CLINIC GUIDE

Cleveland Clinic Press/January 2006

All rights reserved

Copyright © The Cleveland Clinic Foundation

No part of this book may be reproduced in a retrieval system or transmitted in any form or through any method including electronic, photocopying, online download or any other system now known or hereafter invented—except by reviewers, who may quote brief passages in a review to be printed in a newspaper or print or online publication—without express written permission from the Cleveland Clinic Press.

Contact:

Cleveland Clinic Press

9500 Euclid Ave. NA32

Cleveland, OH 44195

216-444-1158

chilnil@ccf.org

www.clevelandclinicpress.org

This book is not intended to replace personal medical care and supervision; there is no substitute for the experience and information that your doctor can provide. Rather, it is our hope that this book will provide additional information to help people understand the nature and diagnosis of arthritis.

Proper medical care should always be tailored to the individual patient. If you read something in this book that seems to conflict with your doctor's instructions, contact your doctor. Since each individual case differs, there will be good reasons for individual treatment to differ from the information presented in this book.

If you have any questions about any treatment in this book, consult your doctor.

The patient names and cases used in this book do not represent actual people, but are composite cases drawn from several sources.

ISBN: 1-59624-008-3

Library of Congress Control Number: 2005933181

Library of Congress Cataloging-in-Publication Data

Clough, John D.

Arthritis: A Cleveland Clinic Guide / by John D. Clough, M.D.

p. cm.

Includes index.

ISBN 1-59624-008-3 (alk. paper)

1. Arthritis—Popular works.   2. Arthritis—Case studies. I. Title.

RC933.C59 2006   616.7'22—dc22

2005029168

Cover and Book Design: Whitney Campbell & Co. • Advertising & Design

Contents

Preface

Almost everybody has, thinks he or she has, or knows someone who has arthritis. Arthritis is a common and thoroughly miserable group of conditions. Statistics from various sources suggest that between 10 and 20 percent of Americans of all ages suffer from some kind of arthritis.

It has been said that there are over one hundred types of arthritis. While that may be something of an exaggeration, it is nonetheless clear that many types exist. Figuring out what type of arthritis a person has carries important implications, both for assessing the risk of disability and for successfully treating that person.

Notwithstanding the wide diversity of arthritic conditions, it is noteworthy that more than 95 percent of arthritis sufferers have one of the ten or so most common types of arthritis, which we review in this book. In addition, we take a look at a couple of very common nonarthritic conditions that are often mistaken for arthritis: fibromyalgia and polymyalgia rheumatica.

One condition that is, perhaps, conspicuous by its absence from this review is Lyme disease, an infection often accompanied by arthritis. Lyme disease occurs in parts of the country where its causative bacterium (*Borrelia burgdorferi*) and carrier (deer tick) are found. Controversy continues to surround this diagnosis, fed by the difficulty in ruling it out definitively in people with nonspecific symptoms of the disease. Some physicians have taken the approach of treating with antibiotics whenever there is even a remote possibility of Lyme disease, while others are purists and require rigorous proof of the diagnosis before treating. Both sides espouse their views with a quasi-religious fervor unwarranted by the data available to them.

Our approach to the common forms of arthritis is to introduce them with stories of hypothetical patients. Although the patients' names are fictitious, their stories are not. Each is based in reality, and the patients' responses to treatment are likewise real. The doctors involved remain mostly unnamed. These are stories about patients, not doctors. But as you read them, remember that every patient is different, and what works for one does not work for all. Nowhere in medicine is the phrase "One man's meat is another man's poison" more relevant than in arthritis. This book may help to point you in the right direction, but it is no substitute for a physician who knows what he or she is doing. The role of the physician is to help you sift through all of the variation and complexity, come to the right conclusions about diagnosis and treatment, and ultimately get as good an outcome as possible.

I wish to acknowledge that I received considerable help in bringing this book to reality. Gloria Mosesson, our consultant, who assisted us a great deal in the early days of the Cleveland Clinic Press, suggested that I write it and gave me a lot of early encouragement. Peter Studer, head of the Cleveland Clinic's Department of Scientific Publications, read every chapter and made many helpful suggestions. Larry Chilnick, the Cleveland Clinic Press's editorial director, pushed me to get it done faster than I ever would have otherwise. Finally, I would like to thank editor Judy Knipe, without whose insightful recommendations this book would be even more over the top than it is already. She tolerated my use of unusual names for the not-so-fictitious patients in most (but not all) cases, but she was totally intolerant of unnecessary medical jargon, and for that I thank her.

John D. Clough, MD

October, 2005

Chapter 1
What's All This About Arthritis?

Do your joints hurt? Are they stiff? Are they swollen? Are they deformed?

Are your muscles weak or sore?

Do you stiffen up after sitting for more than a few minutes?

Are you tired all the time? Do you feel old and decrepit beyond your years?

Do you find yourself eating aspirin or ibuprofen on a regular basis?

Do you have (or think you may have) arthritis?

If the answer to any or all of these questions is yes, you might benefit by considering the following.

What is arthritis?

"Arthritis" is a word with a very specific meaning, unlike the ambiguous term "rheumatism," which to most people means aches and pains in the musculoskeletal system. "Arthritis" means inflammation in one or more joints. Aching and stiffness do not necessarily mean you have arthritis, and by the same token, arthritis isn't just pain in the joints. There must be some additional evidence of inflammation, such as swelling, redness, tenderness, stiffness, or unusual warmth, and it must actually be in the joints, not just in muscles or other tissues around the joints.

Joint pain, which is called arthralgia, in itself doesn't equate to arthritis; nevertheless, arthritis is usually painful. The severity may range from moderate and merely annoying to severe and unbearably excruciating. Pain is seldom completely absent from an inflamed joint if the sensory nerves serving the joint are normal. In most cases of arthritis, pain is the dominant symptom, though not the only one, especially early on. Later, disability may become more important, especially if treatment is delayed.

Although many arthritis sufferers have aching muscles (myalgia) and sore tendons (tendinitis) or bursas (bursitis), these latter maladies are not arthritis. They represent different forms of rheumatism that may or may not occur along with arthritis. What makes arthritis more significant than these other forms of rheumatism—painful though they may be—is the potential of arthritis to lead, in some cases, to joint destruction and permanent disability. Once arthritis has damaged a joint, clearing up the inflammation does not return the joint to a normal state. Accordingly, it is important to recognize arthritis early and treat it aggressively before damage occurs.

Arthritis should not be thought of as a disease, but rather as a symptom that is common to many diseases. When arthritis is the most prominent symptom of the disease it happens to be a part of, the disease is often known as a form of arthritis, as, for example, rheumatoid arthritis, a systemic disease that prominently involves the joints, along with other tissues. But many diseases that feature arthritis as a component are not called arthritis. Systemic lupus erythematosus is a prime example. The majority of people with lupus have arthritis as one symptom, but the disease is not primarily thought of as a form of arthritis, probably because involvement of organs other than the joints—for example, the kidneys and the central nervous system—can be much more serious than joint involvement in lupus.

Are there many kinds of arthritis?

The most common forms of arthritis are rheumatoid arthritis and osteoarthritis. But there are, unfortunately, many other kinds, most of which are not nearly as familiar. This book will examine in some detail several different forms of arthritis and review the distinguishing features of the most common types of arthritic disease.

Arthritis is a common problem. The table below shows that the various forms of arthritis affect more than 25 million people in this country, and some estimates are almost twice that figure.

Arthritis Diagnosis	Number of Americans Affected
Osteoarthritis	21,000,000
Rheumatoid arthritis	2,100,000
Gout	2,100,000
Seronegative spondyloarthropathies *(including ankylosing spondylitis and psoriatic arthritis)*	375,000
Systemic lupus erythematosus	240,000
Juvenile arthritis	40,000

The Centers for Disease Control and Prevention (CDC) estimate that arthritis causes disability for 8 million people. It leads to 750,000 hospitalizations and 9,500 deaths annually. It costs the U.S. economy $51 billion in medical costs and $86 billion in total costs each year. It is clearly an important problem, both medically and economically. But those numbers only hint at the human misery arthritis causes.

In some cases, arthritis is not even the most threatening manifestation of the disease that causes it, although it often demands the greatest attention because of the pain that accompanies it. Arthritis may be the most prominent early manifestation of such varied diseases as lung cancer, systemic lupus erythematosus, hepatitis, rheumatic fever, tuberculosis, AIDS, and a host of other nasty afflictions. Making the right diagnosis and treating the underlying disease offer the best chance of success in managing these types of arthritis. Clues suggesting the correct diagnosis can be found in such simple things as:

- which joints (and how many) are affected

- the length of time and the frequency of joint involvement (intermittent vs. constant, acute vs. gradual onset, and other similar parameters)

- the amount of pain, tenderness, stiffness, and swelling, as well as relevant abnormalities in areas of the body other than the joints—for instance, skin rashes, hair loss, mouth ulcers, fever, nodules under the skin, and other signs and symptoms

Although a skilled physician can usually tell with considerable confidence what is going on from these clues, additional information from the laboratory and X-ray departments may help nail down the diagnosis.

What is the likely outcome of arthritis?

Outcomes vary. The diverse forms of arthritis are, in most cases, chronic conditions for which there are no known cures. Even joint infections successfully treated and cured with antibiotics often leave enough residual damage in the affected joints to be chronically problematic thereafter. So, a "satisfactory" outcome is a relative thing, depending on the type of arthritis, the stage of the disease when treatment is begun, the willingness and ability of the patient to tolerate and persevere in treatment, activity levels, and other health factors.

Establishing appropriate expectations and time frames for the results of treatment is a key component of achieving a satisfactory outcome. If the expectation is that the disease will be cured, with complete relief of all symptoms and no need for long-term medications and medical follow-up, disappointment will be inevitable. Nevertheless, many people with arthritis live happy and productive lives through a combination of understanding and accommodating to the limitations imposed by the disease along with the appropriate use of medical, surgical, and other treatment modalities.

Are there special doctors who treat arthritis?

Normally, the overall treatment programs for people with arthritis should be planned, supervised, and in some cases monitored by specially trained physicians called rheumatologists. Realistically, however, people who develop arthritic symptoms almost always consult an internist or family physician when they first develop symptoms. These primary-care physicians frequently refer patients with arthritis to rheumatologists, both to make or confirm the diagnosis and to suggest or initiate treatment. Although rheumatology is a relatively young specialty, in today's world we can generally expect that, after graduating from medical school, a rheumatologist will have been trained in internal medicine for at least two years, followed by a fellowship in rheumatology for two or three years in an accredited training program. Evidence of successful completion of such training is dual board certification in internal medicine and in rheumatology, generally by the American Board of Internal Medicine or the American Osteopathic Board of Internal Medicine. Some physicians trained in foreign countries may have different qualifications and credentials.

In the United States, approximately 4,000 rheumatologists are currently in active practice, but like many other medical specialists, they are not evenly distributed throughout the country. They tend to concentrate in larger cities and in academic medical centers, although this is not universally true. Many practice in groups, either with other rheumatologists or in groups of other specialists, but many communities have no rheumatologists at all. For individuals living in such communities, frequent hands-on treatment by a rheumatologist is not practical. Fortunately, rheumatologists are trained to work with primary-care physicians, who can supervise and monitor treatment of properly diagnosed patients with care plans.

What treatments are available for arthritis?

Although arthritic diseases can seldom be cured, the good news is that there is treatment, varying in effectiveness, for all of them. Depending on the type and severity of the arthritis, this treatment may run the gamut from mild physical and/or occupational therapy through aggressive chemotherapy and surgery. As we consider the different types of arthritis in this book, we shall review the treatments available for each in some detail, putting them in the context of specific patients, with some attention to the side effects that might be encountered.

Drug treatments

Depending on the type of arthritis being treated, medications include:

• **Anti-inflammatory agents**, ranging from mild and familiar oral medications, such as aspirin, to powerful new medicines that must be given by injection, such as etanercept and infliximab.

• **Immunosuppressive medicines** (drugs that inhibit the immune system) may be prescribed in rheumatoid arthritis, especially when the activity of disease is moderate or severe.

• **Antibiotics** are used in infectious arthritis.

• **Uric acid–lowering agents** are employed to treat gout.

• **Corticosteroids** (cortisone-like drugs) may be effective when injected into the involved joints where only one or two joints are inflamed—a benefit that tends to be temporary, but sometimes is all the treatment that is needed.

The effectiveness of immunosuppressives, antibiotics, and uric acid–lowering drugs depends on the correctness of the diagnosis, while the anti-inflammatory agents are more generally effective.

Generic drug names

In this book, I have chosen to refer to all drugs by their generic names. There are several good reasons to take this approach. In many cases, after the initial patent period expires (by law, twenty years after the drug is invented), different companies market the same drugs under a variety of names. Which brand name would we then use? The same thing may happen when a drug previously requiring a prescription becomes available over the counter (OTC). As an example, ibuprofen by prescription is called Motrin, but the OTC forms include, among others, Advil, Nuprin, and Motrin-OTC.

To add to the confusion, companies may market the same drug under different names in different countries; for instance, indomethacin is Indocin in the United States, but Indocid in many other countries. Moreover, discarded names of withdrawn drugs may be recycled and used for totally different drugs. For example, zomepirac, known as Zomax initially, was withdrawn from the market a decade ago. The name Zomax now refers to one company's brand of azithromycin, a familiar antibiotic, marketed in the United States as Zithromax. We don't need this kind of confusion. Nevertheless, for the sake of convenience, I have listed in appendix B the generic names of the drugs mentioned in the book, along with a selection of brand names current at the time of this writing.

Bringing drugs to market

Since drugs play such an important role in the treatment of most forms of arthritis, it is worth considering, at least briefly, the processes by which these drugs are discovered or invented, tested, approved, and released for general use.

Until fairly recently, most drugs employed in the treatment of arthritis were already in existence for some other indication. Their antiarthritic effects were, for the most part, serendipitously discovered when the drugs were given for another reason to someone who happened to have arthritis, producing an unexpected beneficial effect on the arthritis. Gold salts, for example, were used to treat certain chronic infections, e.g., tuberculosis. Antimalarial drugs were used to prevent or treat malaria. Methotrexate and other chemotherapy drugs were used to treat cancer. Most of these medicines came into widespread use in treating arthritis based on anecdotal experience, without their having undergone rigorous investigation for either effectiveness or safety in arthritis patients. For example, methotrexate treatment for rheumatoid arthritis began in the 1960s, but studies validating its use for this indication were not reported until twenty years later. Patents on such drugs had long since expired by the time the drugs were given to arthritis patients.

More recently, pharmaceutical companies have been making new drugs designed specifically for treating arthritis. These drugs are of two general types. The more common ones are the me-too drugs, based on existing drugs but modified either to achieve greater convenience of administration (e.g., once- or twice-a-day dosing rather than four times a day) or improved safety (e.g., COX-2–inhibiting NSAIDs). The other type includes the truly innovative drugs, like the TNF-alpha inhibitors, which work by novel mechanisms and are clearly more effective than their predecessors.

Both types of new drugs go through extensive prerelease testing for safety (Phase 1) and effectiveness (Phase 2), requiring an average of seven years from the time the drugs are invented. When the data are available, the Food and Drug Administration (FDA) reviews them and makes a determination as to whether the new drug is effective enough and safe enough to be released, so that doctors can prescribe it. There is some urgency to this, because the patent clock starts ticking when the drug is invented, not at the time it is released by the FDA, and once the twenty-year patent has expired, the drug goes into the public domain, where it can be manufactured and sold by anyone who can meet certain FDA standards. Thus, the company that bore the entire risk and considerable cost associated with developing and testing the new drug no longer has exclusive rights to it.

Given these pressures, it becomes somewhat easier to understand how some relatively uncommon side effects of a new drug might not be recognized during the prerelease testing phases. When recognition of such side effects eventually does occur, there is often pressure to force withdrawal of the drug in question, sometimes accompanied by accusations of duplicitous suppression of negative data by the manufacturer (which unfortunately has occasionally turned out to be true).

Surgical treatments

Surgical treatments, carried out by orthopedic surgeons, are indicated to repair or reconstruct some damaged joints that are painful or causing disability because they are no longer mechanically functional. Progress in joint replacement technology applicable to large weight-bearing joints—hips and knees—has been dramatic over the past three decades, and highly satisfactory results are now commonplace. In some cases, shoulder or elbow replacement can give good results as well. Wrist and ankle replacement are more problematic, but this technology is developing. Lesser procedures are also appropriate in some cases.

Physical and occupational therapy

Physical and occupational therapy have an important place in the treatment of arthritis. Passive modalities, such as application of heat, and active strengthening and range-of-motion exercises also offer benefits to many patients. Because of the differing needs of patients with different forms of arthritis or in different stages of any form of arthritis, these therapy programs need to be individually designed and supervised by trained individuals who understand the diseases and know what they are doing. These include physiatrists (specialists in physical medicine and rehabilitation, not to be confused with psychiatrists), physical therapists, and occupational therapists.

Treatment for depression

Arthritis, being a chronic, unrelenting problem, also takes an emotional toll that can seriously tax a person's normal coping mechanisms. Depression is a frequent and not unexpected outcome of arthritis that needs to be dealt with as it becomes evident. Not everybody with arthritis needs to see a psychiatrist or a psychologist, but some do. In addition, the disease affects families—spouses and children—of patients. It puts stress on marriages, drains finances, and limits productivity. Marital and family counseling may be needed.

Chapter 2
Rheumatoid Arthritis

Onset: The nightmare begins

Life was good for Beulah. She was an attractive twenty-three-year-old executive secretary, happily married for one year, and had just begun thinking about starting a family. Her husband, Clifford, three years older than she, was an engineer with an excellent future in the aerospace industry. They met at a college mixer, began dating, and then married right after they both graduated. They seemed to be the perfect couple—young, in love, and living the American dream, with their future bright before them. Then, without warning, their world gradually began to collapse into a nightmare.

One day, Clifford noticed a small lump in his neck. It wasn't sore, so he ignored it. But the lump didn't go away, and when he realized it was gradually getting bigger, he consulted his physician to see what the problem was. The lump was a lymph node, and the biopsy diagnosis was non-Hodgkin's lymphoma, a nasty, malignant disease of the lymphatic system.

Over the next few months, despite aggressive treatment, Clifford got sicker and sicker. His spleen and liver were affected. He lost forty pounds. It was hard to tell which made him more miserable—the disease or the treatment. Soon it became clear that Clifford wasn't going to make it. Beulah was beside herself with worry. Although she tried to act brave around Clifford, she was devastated emotionally and, to an increasing extent, physically.

Shortly after Clifford's diagnosis, Beulah began to feel stiff, particularly in her hands and wrists, and she noticed some puffiness in these regions. *Figure 1.* Soon the symptoms spread to her shoulders, elbows, hips, knees, ankles, and feet. Her jaw joints were painful, and her voice became hoarse. As Clifford progressively went downhill, so did Beulah, although she tried to conceal her discomfort when she was around him. But she

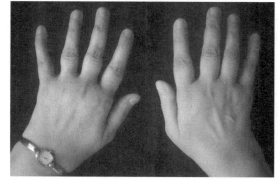

Figure 1: Hands of a person with early, as yet nondestructive rheumatoid arthritis. The same joints are affected in both hands (symmetrical), and the distal joints of the fingers (most distant from the wrists) are usually spared.

had increasing difficulty carrying out simple tasks—opening jars, turning faucets on and off, and typing. She was taking large doses of aspirin, which gave her some relief, but her stomach was rebelling against this abuse. She was so focused on her husband's plight that she didn't take proper care of her own worsening problems.

Clifford died almost six months to the day after having been diagnosed. By then, Beulah was so disabled that she could hardly get through the wake and the funeral. She really became scared when she noticed some lumps under her skin, just below the elbows. *Figure 2*. The lumps weren't sore, just as Clifford's first swollen lymph node had been pain free. As soon as Clifford was buried, Beulah scheduled an appointment with her internist to find out what her problem was. After an examination and some tests, he sat down with her to discuss the findings.

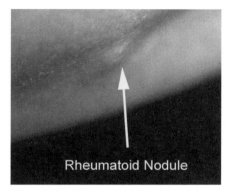
Rheumatoid Nodule

Figure 2: Small rheumatoid nodule located just below the elbow. This is a typical location, but nodules may be found in many other sites as well.

How did the doctor know the diagnosis?

"Beulah, it seems pretty clear that you've developed rheumatoid arthritis," her doctor began. "Your story is fairly typical for the way rheumatoid arthritis often begins: onset of pain, stiffness, and swelling in many joints, especially the small joints of the hands, wrists, and the jaw [temporomandibular] in a young woman, often preceded by a traumatic event. I strongly suspected the diagnosis as soon as I heard that much of your story.

"We were able to confirm the diagnosis by noting that the distribution of the joints affected was mostly symmetrical—meaning the same joints are involved on both sides—and that the lumps below your elbows were typical rheumatoid nodules, that is, firm, spherical, nontender masses of tissue under the skin, about a half-inch in diameter. I also suspect that your hoarseness might be caused by arthritis of the joints in the voice box. This is fairly common in rheumatoid arthritis.

"Your blood tests showed mild anemia, and tests for inflammatory activity—sedimentation rate and C-reactive protein—were elevated. In addition, there is an abnormal antibody in your blood called rheumatoid factor. This is an autoantibody directed against IgG, a normal blood protein. An antibody that reacts against components of one's own body is called an autoantibody. Rheumatoid factor is typically present in people with rheumatoid arthritis, occurring in about 80 percent of those with this disease, but it is also often found in several other conditions as well as in some older people without any apparent disease."

The doctor concluded, "I would like you to see a colleague of mine, a specialist in rheumatology, who is experienced in the diagnosis and treatment of rheumatoid arthritis. If that's okay with you, I'll ask my secretary to set up the appointment."

Beulah readily gave her consent, and when she arrived at the rheumatologist's office a few days later, he continued the conversation begun by the internist.

"I've reviewed the X-rays of your chest, hands, and wrists," the rheumatologist said. "The hand films showed no erosions around the small joints typical of destructive rheumatoid arthritis, but there did appear to be some calcium loss in the bones adjacent to the joints, a condition called juxta-articular osteoporosis, which is often seen in early stages of the disease. Your wrists had similar calcium loss, but there were no erosions there, either. This indicates that, so far at least, there's not a lot of destruction due to the disease." *Figure 3.*

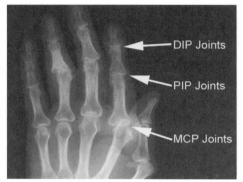

Figure 3: X-ray of the hand of a patient with destructive rheumatoid arthritis. Several of the PIP (proximal interphalangeal) and MCP (metacarpophalangeal) joints are damaged, but the DIP (distal interphalangeal) joints are spared.

"In the chest X-ray, your internist and I were looking for several things, none of which, fortunately, was present. Sometimes an inflammatory form of arthritis is the earliest sign of cancer, especially lung cancer. Some people with true rheumatoid arthritis get rheumatoid nodules—like those you have at your elbows—in the lungs, where they look very similar to cancer on an X-ray. Rheumatoid arthritis can be associated with other chest X-ray findings as well, including an accumulation of fluid around the lungs—known as pleural effusion—or fibrotic changes in the lung tissue. A few people with tuberculosis and other uncommon infectious diseases get arthritis as a symptom. But as it turned out, your chest X-ray was clear.

"Based on all this information," the rheumatologist said, "I agree with the diagnosis of rheumatoid arthritis, and we are now able to begin mapping out a course of treatment for you."

Beulah listened attentively and then began asking questions.

What causes rheumatoid arthritis? Did I "catch" this disease?

The doctor answered, "We don't know what causes rheumatoid arthritis, despite years of research. It's one of the autoimmune diseases, in the sense that immune mechanisms that normally protect us from infections and malignancies somehow become misdirected so as to attack components of our own bodies. These mechanisms cause inflammation in various tissues, most characteristically the joint-lining tissues, called the synovial membranes. This inflammation is ultimately destructive if it isn't controlled.

"Among the suggested possible causes of rheumatoid arthritis is infection. Some infections are known to be able to activate the immune system to cause autoimmune damage. An example is a particular strain of streptococcus, a common cause of sore throat that can lead to rheumatic fever or acute kidney disease by inducing inappropriate, self-destructive immune activity. Although great efforts have been expended in trying to identify such a cause for rheumatoid arthritis, it hasn't been possible to do so. There's no convincing evidence that a person can 'catch' rheumatoid arthritis from someone else."

What was the role of the traumatic event—Clifford's illness and death?

"The relationship between acute stress and immune function has been the subject of some investigation and a lot of speculation," the doctor replied. "Some studies have suggested that hormones originating in the nervous system—neurohormones, if you will—play an important role in regulating immune function. These systems can be perturbed by stress, whether emotional or physical. Many believe that such a mechanism may underlie the frequent observation that autoimmune diseases, especially rheumatoid arthritis, appear to be triggered or aggravated by stressors. The list of the top ten emotional stressors first reported by U.S. navy physicians Thomas Holmes and Richard Rahe in 1967—and now known as the Holmes-Rahe Scale—is headed by death of a spouse."

The rheumatologist continued, "Although the cause is unknown, there are some peculiar features of the disease that are probably clues to its cause, if only we knew how to interpret them. For instance, there is evidence from the study of ancient human remains that rheumatoid arthritis appeared relatively recently in our history;

before AD 1500, there is no evidence that the disease existed in the Old World, but Native American populations may have been affected earlier. Statements in the older medical literature to the effect that examinations of ancient Egyptian skeletons revealed evidence of rheumatoid arthritis have been superseded by the more recent recognition that the abnormalities seen there were due to ankylosing spondylitis, not rheumatoid arthritis. Rheumatoid arthritis is about three times more frequent in women than in men. There are two peaks in age of onset, the first relatively early—fifteen to thirty-five years of age—and the other relatively late—after age seventy. How all these seemingly disparate facts could be related continues to elude explanation.

"In addition, there is a genetic aspect to rheumatoid arthritis. The disease is more common in people who have a family history of rheumatoid arthritis, and there is an association with certain inherited blood cell antigens known as HLA antigens. This association acts as a susceptibility factor rather than a direct link to the cause of the disease. Any of the rheumatoid patient's children who inherit the susceptibility factor have an increased likelihood of getting the disease. That does not mean that they will surely get the disease or that children without the antigen won't get it, but it does affect the odds."

"Well," Beulah said, "the practical question for me is, what do I have to look forward to in the way of disability?"

Will I be crippled?

"Our job is to try to prevent that, but only time can truly answer your question," responded the doctor. "In some cases, the disease is mild and responds to minimal treatment. In others, it is hard to control and very aggressive, attacking not only the joints but many other tissues as well, including the small blood vessels, eyes, lungs, and heart. Most of the time, however, the disease smolders along relentlessly, and unless it can be controlled, over time it can do a lot of damage to the joints.

"Treatment for rheumatoid arthritis improved dramatically during the last quarter of the twentieth century, and there is now evidence that some medications can slow or prevent joint damage in many people with the disease, assuming that they can tolerate the medications. Such drugs are often referred to as DMARDs, or disease-modifying antirheumatic drugs. Once damage has occurred, however, medications can't reverse it, but surgical reconstructive procedures have much more to offer now than in the past."

"Does the fact that I have rheumatoid arthritis make me more susceptible to other problems?" asked Beulah.

Does rheumatoid arthritis or its treatment predispose me to other diseases?

"That is a very good question," said the rheumatologist. "Rheumatoid arthritis is sometimes complicated by other autoimmune diseases."

Sjögren's syndrome

"Sjögren's syndrome is named after a famous Swedish eye surgeon who first recognized it in the early 1930s," the doctor told Beulah. "In this condition, the eyes and mouth are very dry because of autoimmune destruction of the salivary glands and the tear, or lacrimal, glands. The disease may attack endocrine glands, such as the thyroid, as well. In Sjögren's syndrome, the immune abnormality is often more profound than in rheumatoid arthritis alone, and this leads to an increased incidence of certain malignancies, including especially lymphoma, myeloma, and leukemia."

Carpal tunnel syndrome

"In people who spend many hours a day working at a computer keyboard, carpal tunnel syndrome is fairly common and believed to be due to repetitive trauma," the doctor said. "But it can also be a complication of inflammation and swelling at the wrist in rheumatoid arthritis. In carpal tunnel syndrome, the median nerve—the main nerve that supplies the thumb, index finger, and part of the third finger—becomes entrapped and compressed at the wrist, leading to pain and tingling in these fingers while sparing the ring finger and the fifth finger. If untreated, permanent damage to the nerve can result, leading to loss of muscle mass in the thenar eminence, the large muscle at the base of the thumb. Other nerve entrapment syndromes are less common, but they can also occur in rheumatoid arthritis."

Amyloidosis

"Amyloidosis is a term used to describe deposits of amorphous—that is, unstructured—tissue in various organs. It's a complication of active rheumatoid arthritis and other chronic inflammatory diseases that remain uncontrolled over a long period of time," the doctor explained. "In some parts of the body it is nothing more than a nuisance, but in the kidneys or the muscles, especially the heart muscle, amyloidosis can become life threatening by interfering with organ function. It's better to control the arthritis adequately up front, in the hope of avoiding amyloidosis, than to try to treat it once it has occurred.

"Other relatively uncommon complications of rheumatoid arthritis include **blood vessel inflammation** (vasculitis) and **eye inflammation** (scleritis and scleromalacia). With modern drug treatment, we seldom encounter such problems these days.

"The treatment of rheumatoid arthritis employs a number of potentially toxic drugs that need to be monitored closely. We'll talk about this a lot more when we get into management of the disease. At this point, it's enough to say that drug toxicity is a big worry. It's a worry from the standpoint of what we know about the drugs that have been in use for many years, as well as what we don't know about the long-term hazards of the more recently introduced drugs. The latter drugs are increasingly used because of their outstanding effectiveness."

"Clifford and I always wanted to have children someday," Beulah said hesitantly. "Now that he's gone, that's out of the question. But with this disease, if I should want to have children in the future, will I be able to? And how likely are they to get rheumatoid arthritis?"

Will I ever be able to have children?
Will they get rheumatoid arthritis?

"Rheumatoid arthritis, in itself, is not known to interfere with fertility," the doctor replied. "But many of the drugs used to treat the disease are potentially hazardous to the developing child during pregnancy, and some of these medications can make conception difficult or impossible, at least while they are being taken. Interestingly, pregnancy may have a beneficial, possibly drug-sparing effect on rheumatoid disease activity, allowing reduction in dosage or even elimination of one or more drugs, so an unintended pregnancy is not necessarily a disaster. But despite that, it's better not to become pregnant while on antirheumatic drug therapy.

"As I mentioned earlier, the disease is more common in people who have a family history of rheumatoid arthritis, especially those with the HLA antigen called DR4. This association is not strong enough to make it necessary to test you to see if you have it, but any of your children who inherit the HLA-DR4 susceptibility factor would have a slightly increased risk of getting the disease."

"I have heard different people say you should exercise or you shouldn't exercise when you have arthritis," recalled Beulah. "Which is it?"

Should I exercise?

The rheumatologist replied, "One of the biggest problems for people with arthritis, whether it is rheumatoid or some other form of arthritis, is that painful joints tend to make a person less active. However, inactivity sets up a vicious cycle in which the inactivity leads to muscle wasting, which in turn leads to decreased strength and even less activity, until a person becomes completely disabled. And inactivity also promotes weight gain, another big problem. Needless to say, this is not good.

"On the other hand, certain kinds of activity can be destructive to joints that may already have some damage from the arthritis. Generally, high-impact exercises, such as running, are to be avoided. Walking is good exercise for most people with arthritis, and swimming is even better. Specific exercise programs should be designed by experts in physical medicine in order to minimize the likelihood of causing damage to joints and tendons."

"I'm a believer in healthy nutrition," said Beulah. "Is there a diet I can follow that will help my arthritis?"

Does diet help?

The rheumatologist was warming to the topic and said, "We live in the age of organic nutrition and alternative therapies, and some people believe that proper nutrition can take care of almost any problem. However, with all due respect to those who like the 'natural' approach to treating disease—to the exclusion of effective medications—this is a formula for disaster in rheumatoid arthritis. The only such treatment for which there is even a modicum of supportive data is the ingestion of fish oil for its anti-inflammatory activity. Although large statistical studies show that arthritic patients on a diet high in fish oil do a little better than those on no special diet, the amount of benefit is small, and the amount of oil needed to achieve it is formidable, to say the least. In Europe and Australia, there are advocates of gluten-free diets, avoidance of chocolate and red meat, and other dietary interventions for which there is little evidence of efficacy.

"To my mind, **the best advice about diet for a patient with arthritis is: Don't get fat.** Carrying excess weight around is a sure way to pulverize your arthritic knees into oblivion. Moderation in eating and judicious exercise are key to keeping your weight in check. Starvation dieting won't work because you must take the noxious antirheumatic medications with food, and marathon running is not an option for most people with arthritis."

"Okay, we've talked about diet and exercise. What about medications?" asked Beulah.

How can we treat this disease?

Beulah's rheumatologist said there was some good news and that modern medications have much to offer. Because Beulah had seropositive (positive rheumatoid factor) arthritis with rheumatoid nodules and multiple joints involved—all indicators of potentially destructive disease—he recommended starting treatment with three basic medications:

• A nonsteroidal anti-inflammatory (aspirin-like) drug, or NSAID (pronounced EN-sed). NSAIDs work by inhibiting cyclooxygenases (COXs), a group of enzymes important in the body's production of an important class of mediators of inflammation, the prostaglandins. The doctor picked **naproxen** for several reasons. Beulah had no history of peptic ulcer disease, liver disease, or kidney disease. An alternative, if she'd had a history of ulcers, might have been one of the new COX-2 inhibitors, which are designed to spare the stomach lining, but these drugs have an uncertain future because they appear to cause coronary artery disease. In addition, the COX-2 inhibitors are expensive, and they have no advantage over the more common NSAIDs in people not prone to ulcers. Naproxen also has the virtues of twice-a-day dosing, reasonable effectiveness, and relatively low cost. The doctor told Beulah to take the drug with food so as not to unduly risk causing her first peptic ulcer. He also mentioned that naproxen would become fully effective within about ten days or two weeks, although there might be some almost immediate benefit.

• **An antimalarial drug.** The effectiveness of this class of drugs in rheumatoid arthritis was one of the circumstantial bits of evidence that suggested an infectious cause for rheumatoid arthritis in the 1950s. Now everyone admits that the reason for the effectiveness of antimalarials is not clear. If you ask a rheumatologist how these drugs work, he or she will likely mumble something about "stabilizing the lysosomes" and rapidly change the subject.

Beulah's doctor chose **hydroxychloroquine** for this purpose, to be taken twice a day. He explained that this drug had several side effects, the most important and dramatic (though rarest) of which is blindness. That got her attention, and she questioned him sharply about hydroxychloroquine. He reassured her that she could take it safely for as long as necessary if (a) she did not exceed the recommended daily dose and (b) she had her eyes examined annually by an ophthalmologist to ascertain that none of the drug's toxic effects on the light-sensitive layer of the eye were present. He also told her that hydroxychloroquine would not reach full effectiveness for at least two months, possibly three.

• **An antimetabolic medication.** Although there are a couple of choices here, Beulah's doctor chose **methotrexate**, a chemotherapy drug that inhibits the body's utilization of the B vitamin folic acid. This vitamin is important in DNA synthesis, which lies at the heart of cell reproduction. Thus, methotrexate preferentially inhibits replication of the most rapidly dividing cell populations, which in active rheumatoid arthritis are the cells in the inflamed areas.

Although methotrexate has been around since the early 1960s, its widespread use in rheumatoid arthritis did not begin until the mid-1980s. By then, the medical profession had become convinced that methotrexate was unique among chemotherapeutic drugs in that it did not materially increase the risk of developing cancer. Beulah's rheumatologist told her that methotrexate could be taken safely as long as it was monitored by blood counts and liver function tests at about three-month intervals. He recommended a starting dose of three tablets weekly and noted that it would take six to twelve weeks for the drug to achieve full effectiveness.

The doctor went on to say, "Because the main drugs that will eventually control the disease won't be effective for weeks to months, you might get some immediate relief from an **injection of a corticosteroid medication**." Beulah agreed to this, and he gave her the injection at once.

Beulah's doctor chose the initial treatment from a larger array of possibilities. He could have started with the antimalarial and the NSAID, planning to add methotrexate later if needed. Because of the time frame in which these drugs work, however, he would have had to wait at least two months before starting methotrexate. He felt strongly, based on the initial severity of Beulah's arthritis, that methotrexate would be needed, and he didn't want to allow the disease to remain active for that length of time, during which a lot of damage could occur.

He explained, "Methotrexate is one of the DMARDs (disease-modifying anti-rheumatic drugs) I referred to earlier. These drugs are thought, or in some cases have been proven, to modify the course of rheumatoid arthritis in some patients, delaying and perhaps preventing erosion formation in the affected joints. Other DMARDs include injectable and oral gold, d-penicillamine, azathioprine, leflunomide, and sulfasalazine. Although these drugs are effective in some patients, compared with methotrexate they are either more toxic or less effective, or both. Some can be used along with methotrexate in very severe cases. They are also slow acting, in most cases slower than methotrexate. Our strategy is to hold them in reserve in case you have an unacceptable response to methotrexate."

Beulah's rheumatologist also considered the advisability of starting her on low-dose chronic prednisone along with the other three drugs. Prednisone is a synthetic cortisone-like drug that has been available for many years. It works fast and provides pretty good symptomatic relief, at least initially, for most patients. He decided against this as a first-line approach in her case because of the side effects of long-term prednisone therapy, especially its tendency to cause osteoporosis, even in low doses. Once started, prednisone is very difficult to discontinue, because it suppresses the body's ability to make its own cortisone and causes atrophy of the adrenal glands, the physiologic source of cortisone.

Response to treatment

With some trepidation, Beulah consented to the proposed treatment, received her corticosteroid injection, and started the three drugs. By the next day, she felt almost normal. Her symptoms had miraculously cleared, as her doctor had predicted. This was the effect of the corticosteroid injection, but he had warned her that this would be temporary and that she needed to take her other medications in order to maintain the benefit.

A week or so later, Beulah noticed that her vision was blurry. The eye toxicity of the antimalarial drug immediately came to her mind, and she called her doctor. He reassured her that although this was most likely a side effect of the antimalarial drug, it was not the serious retinal toxicity, but rather was related to hydroxychloroquine's tendency to cause relaxation of the small muscles in the eye that focus the lens. This is normally a temporary effect and clears without the need to stop the drug, and that was the case with Beulah.

Over the next few weeks, some of her arthritic symptoms gradually recurred, but not as severely as before treatment. Beulah felt well enough to return to work, and as the weeks went by and the long-acting drugs became effective, most of her symptoms again subsided. Her only problem was chronic mild inflammation in the right wrist, which eventually led to loss of motion in this joint. She followed the testing regimen scheduled by her doctor, including annual eye examinations and blood tests every three months, and had no further problems for the next couple of years.

Then one day, she began to have irregular vaginal bleeding. She consulted her gynecologist, who tried several approaches, including a dilatation and curettage (D and C), with no benefit. The gynecologist suspected that methotrexate might be the culprit and recommended that this be discontinued. With the concurrence of her rheumatologist, Beulah stopped methotrexate, and the bleeding subsided almost immediately.

Over the next few weeks, however, her arthritis became more active in multiple joints, especially the right wrist. After a second trial of methotrexate, which controlled the arthritis but again caused vaginal bleeding, it was clear that Beulah was not going to be able to use methotrexate for her arthritis. But she needed something to achieve an acceptable level of control of the disease.

New drugs and further choices

When a previously effective medication regimen for rheumatoid arthritis loses its effectiveness or has to be discontinued because of side effects, several choices have to be made, depending on the circumstances. If the problem is loss of effectiveness, sometimes the solution is simply to increase the dose. There are limits to this approach, since the risk of side effects generally increases as the dose is increased. Obviously, this was not the solution to Beulah's problem, as she already had experienced an intolerable side effect of methotrexate.

In seeking a replacement for methotrexate, one possible choice would have been to try one of the other DMARDs previously mentioned. Since the onset of Beulah's illness, however, some new, highly effective drugs had become available. The FDA had approved a new class of apparently safe medications for use in rheumatoid arthritis. These drugs were inhibitors of a potent inflammatory mediator called **tumor necrosis factor-alpha (TNF-alpha)**. TNF-alpha is one of the intercellular mediators collectively known as **cytokines**. Nevertheless, enthusiasm for the use of TNF-alpha inhibitors was tempered by several facts. It was worrisome that nothing was known of the long-term toxicity of these agents, since they had been in use only since 1998. Furthermore, they could not be taken orally but had to be administered only by injection. In addition, they were extremely expensive. Finally, their availability was initially limited by the manufacturer's low production capacity, although this problem was soon corrected. Despite these drawbacks, Beulah's rheumatologist felt that a TNF-alpha inhibitor might be the best solution to her current dilemma because of the known toxicity and uncertain effectiveness of the older medications. He began the application process with her insurance company to get preauthorization to start her on **etanercept**, the first of the TNF-alpha inhibitors approved for use in rheumatoid arthritis.

Beulah eventually obtained a supply of etanercept and learned to inject herself with it weekly, rotating among several injection sites as she had been instructed. Within a few weeks, she had an excellent response to etanercept and for all intents and purposes felt normal for the first time since the onset of her arthritis. She was only slightly limited by the damage to her right wrist and continued to do well for at least three years thereafter.

Etanercept is not the only TNF-alpha inhibitor currently available and FDA approved for treatment of rheumatoid arthritis. Others are **infliximab**, previously approved for use in inflammatory bowel disease, and **adalimumab.** All are quite effective. They differ somewhat in the route and frequency of administration, but all must be injected. Etanercept is a genetically engineered, synthetic receptor for TNF-alpha, and infliximab and adalimumab are monoclonal antibodies that bind TNF-alpha. In looking at the generic names of these drugs, the suffix "-mab" is a clue that the drug in question is a monoclonal antibody (see appendix C, the glossary, for a definition).

Inhibitors of other cytokines may also be helpful in rheumatoid arthritis. **Anakinra,** for example, is an **interleukin-1** (IL-1) inhibitor that the FDA has approved for use in rheumatoid arthritis. IL-1 is another cytokine important in inflammation. Anakinra's early record for safety has also been good. These new treatments are products of recombinant DNA technology. It is likely that this technology will provide us with many additional new drugs over the next few years.

What lies in store?

Beulah has rheumatoid arthritis, which, as we have noted, is a chronic disease of unknown cause for which there is no known cure. As of this writing, she has had the disease for seven years. Although she is doing well now, the disease has caused some permanent damage to her right wrist, and the potential for more damage exists. Her body has rejected one effective treatment (methotrexate), and it may reject others. As yet unknown long-term side effects of her medications may emerge.

Beulah may eventually need surgery to reconstruct damaged joints. At present, wrist replacement surgery has not yet come of age, but very good options exist for the hips, knees, shoulders, and elbows.

Although Beulah's course can be viewed as an example of how things may go in rheumatoid arthritis, every patient is different. Now there are few clues that allow us to predict how an individual patient will respond to any treatment for the disease. Results from the Human Genome Project may someday allow individualization of treatment with much less of the trial-and-error approach that Beulah and other patients now have to go through. Beulah's menstrual abnormalities, for example, are an unusual complication of methotrexate treatment, but she hasn't (as yet) had any of the more common complications (liver function abnormalities, suppression of the bone marrow, nausea, hair loss, pneumonitis).

Beulah is a "good" patient. She is bright and communicative, and her doctor appreciates her thoughtful participation in her own care. She makes an effort to understand what her body is telling her and what the potentials and limitations of her treatment are. She has a good sense of humor and supportive people around her. All of these characteristics work to her benefit and will help to assure the best outcome possible, given her circumstances and the available technology.

Disease at a glance: Rheumatoid arthritis

Who gets it?

- Most frequent onset in women of child-bearing age
- Weak heredity component
- 2.1 million Americans affected

Joint involvement

- Generally polyarticular (involving multiple joints)
- Symmetrical joint involvement
- Prominent erosions and joint destruction

Other features and complications

- Rheumatoid nodules
- Vasculitis
- Sjögren's syndrome
- Scleritis and scleromalacia
- Amyloidosis

Laboratory features

- Rheumatoid factor in 80 percent
- Elevated acute phase reactants (e.g., sedimentation rate, CRP)

Treatment

- General
    - o Adequate rest
    - o Appropriate exercise
    - o Education
- Medications
    - o Aspirin or other NSAID
    - o Antimalarial drug
    - o Methotrexate and/or other DMARD
    - o TNF-alpha inhibitor
    - o Local joint injections
- Surgery if appropriate

Chapter 3

Osteoarthritis

Onset: I must be getting old!

It was morning of the first day of Harry's retirement. For almost everybody else, Monday was a workday, but not for Harry. Not any longer. He luxuriated in sleeping in, which for him meant not getting up until 6:30 a.m. He was looking forward to working in the yard that day, and it looked as though the weather was going to cooperate. The sun was out, and the birds were singing. Through the open window, he could hear the dull roar of the interstate a mile or so away and pictured himself somewhat wistfully on the road heading for the office, but he soon put that out of his mind and refocused his attention on getting out of bed and getting dressed. Stella, his wife, was already up and puttering around in the kitchen. Although she might have been a little jittery about having him around all the time, Harry was determined not to make a pest of himself. No, he would just have his breakfast, especially the two cups of black coffee he always drank, read the paper, and go outdoors to start mowing the grass, a job he had "outsourced" for the last ten years.

As Harry headed for the shower, the stiffness that had been minimally bothering him for a few minutes each morning for the last several months began to clear, and the accustomed ache in his left groin began to improve as well. The shower and shave revived him still further, and by the time he strolled into the kitchen in his jeans and work shirt, he was cheerful and ready for action.

"Mornin', Stell," he chirped.

"Yeah," she replied, without looking up from a piecrust she was rolling out. Stella was not a morning person.

"Guess I'll have some bacon and eggs for breakfast."

"They're in the fridge. Help yourself, but don't make a mess," Stella said.

"I don't want to get in the way," Harry offered gamely.

"Better not," she snorted.

This was not going the way he'd expected. He thought Stella might show a little respect for his long career and the hard work he had done to support her while she stayed at home, took care of the house, and looked after the kids. However, she looked unimpressed and didn't appear at all eager to fix him some bacon and eggs.

Although Harry knew that Stella wasn't a morning person, this was a little unusual, even for her. He wondered what he had done wrong and decided to try for a little sympathy.

"Hip hurts this morning," he noted.

"Too bad. My knee hurts, but you don't hear me moaning and groaning about it. It's all swollen up, too," Stella said, one-upping him as she finally looked him in the eye. "Been that way for a month. Hands hurt, too."

"Sorry. I didn't know you were having a problem. Maybe we ought to go see the doctor," Harry suggested. "Kill two birds with one stone."

"Yeah, I guess," Stella said, washing her hands. "Let's go."

"But I haven't had my breakfast yet," Harry complained.

"Eat later. Let's go," Stella said without sympathy.

On the way to the doctor's office, Harry made another try at conversation.

"How long have your joints been hurting, Stell?"

"Ten years."

Harry was a little sheepish about not having noticed her affliction. In fact, there had not been an overabundance of communication between them in recent years, what with his preoccupation with his job and her tendency toward stoicism.

"Why didn't you say something about it?"

"Didn't know you were interested," Stella said. "Anyway, it's just arthritis. Can't do anything about it," she added, although she was on her way to try to do just that.

They rode the rest of the way in silence. Soon after their arrival at the doctor's office, the doctor questioned and examined both of them and ordered some blood tests and X-rays. Before they went to have these studies completed, however, he told them that he believed they both probably had osteoarthritis, and that Stella might be a candidate for surgery on her knee.

On their way down to X-ray, Harry said, "Looks like we have more in common than I thought."

Stella ruefully replied, "Ain't that a kick in the head?"

How did the doctor know the diagnosis?

At sixty years of age, Stella had always enjoyed good health, though she really did not make much of an effort to take care of herself. She was fifteen pounds overweight and did not exercise, although she worked around the house incessantly, both inside and out. When she was about fifty, she began to notice deformities of the distal (outermost) joints of the fingers, just like those her mother and older sister had. *Figure 1.* These bony bumps were red and tender when they first appeared, but they gradually became less inflamed. Although they ached when the weather was cold and wet, mostly they were just unsightly and not much of an impediment to the function of her hands. When Stella was fifty-five, she began to have some intermittent aching in the right knee, which hadn't bothered her since she twisted it taking a spill on the ice in her mid-twenties. It had swollen up

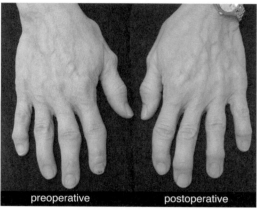

preoperative   postoperative

Figure 1: Bony enlargements at the DIP (distal interphalangeal) joints of a patient with osteoarthritis are called Heberden's nodes. In some patients such enlargements are present at the PIP (proximal interphalangeal) joints, where they are called Bouchard's nodes. The Heberden's nodes on the right hand (shown on left) have been surgically removed, while those on the other hand are still present. Surgical removal of these enlargements is usually not necessary.

then for a few days, but the swelling had gone down, leaving her with no symptoms except occasional clicking of the knee when she stretched it out after a period of inactivity. By the time she was fifty-seven, the right knee was always painful when she

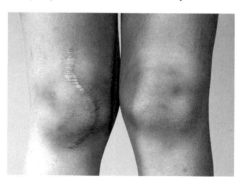

Figure 2: Knock-knee (valgus) deformity, characteristic of osteoarthritis with loss of cartilage in the lateral compartments of the knees.

shifted her weight to that leg. Lately, Stella had begun to notice swelling of the knee, worse at some times than at others but always present. In addition, the knee felt unstable, and when she looked in the mirror, she noticed that her right leg was developing a knock-kneed appearance. *Figure 2.* The doctor told her that this was called a valgus deformity, that it was common in osteoarthritis of the knee, and that it was often, as in Stella's case, accompanied by instability of the joint with a tendency for the knee to give way.

Harry's health had also been good throughout his life. Unlike Stella, he took some pride in looking after himself. He was careful about what he ate, and he exercised regularly on a treadmill, even though it aggravated his left groin pain. He had supplemented his diet with daily vitamin C ever since he'd heard that Linus Pauling, the famous physicist, recommended vitamin C to strengthen the immune response and prevent colds. Harry had regular physical examinations, knew his cholesterol level, and hadn't smoked in many years, so he was somewhat surprised to learn that his groin discomfort might indicate the presence of osteoarthritis of the hip. The doctor told him that his left leg measured a little shorter than the right and that the range of motion of the left hip was somewhat restricted as compared with the right. He also said that the most common symptom of osteoarthritis of the hip was groin pain and that lateral hip pain or buttock pain did not usually originate in the hip joint itself.

For both Stella and Harry, the diagnosis of osteoarthritis was confirmed by X-ray. Stella had almost no cartilage left in the lateral compartment of the right knee, resulting in the knock-kneed appearance and the instability of the knee. *Figure 3*. Although Stella had no X-rays of her hands, the doctor told her that the abnormal process in her hands was osteoarthritis as well. Harry had also lost significant cartilage at the upper part of the left hip, making the joint "space" appear narrow as compared with the other side. Blood tests were normal for both Stella and Harry, as is generally the case in osteoarthritis.

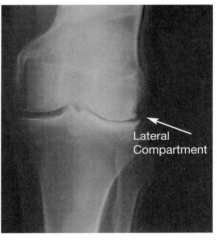

Figure 3: X-ray showing loss of joint "space" (actually cartilage) in the lateral compartment of the left knee in a patient with advanced osteoarthritis. The joint cartilage in the medial compartment is reasonably well preserved.

At the summation visit with their physician, after hearing the diagnosis and findings, Harry and Stella began to ask their questions.

Stella went first. "What did we do to get osteoarthritis? Can you tell what caused it?"

What causes osteoarthritis?

Their doctor responded, "As with most forms of arthritis, the exact cause of osteoarthritis is unknown. Unlike rheumatoid arthritis, which is an inflammatory condition of the joint membrane, or synovium, osteoarthritis is a degenerative condition of the joint cartilage, the shock-absorbing cushion of gristle that is found in all joints. While in rheumatoid arthritis the primary abnormality is inflammation, in osteoarthritis inflammation occurs secondary to mechanical irritation of the degenerated joint. An osteoarthritic joint is not necessarily inflamed, and therefore, the name is something of a misnomer. The British call it osteoarthrosis to indicate that it is not basically an inflammatory condition.

"Although we really don't know the cause," the doctor continued, "we do know about some predisposing factors:

"**Advancing age is one factor.** Scientists think that the joint cartilage may contain less fluid in older individuals and may become brittle and develop tiny cracks, leading to deterioration of the cartilages that cushion the joints.

"**Another possible factor is previous injury** or damage to a joint, even injury caused by a disease like rheumatoid arthritis, which can have secondary osteoarthritis superimposed upon it." Looking at Stella, the doctor went on. "It is possible that your knee injury many years before may have produced a minimal degree of damage to the knee cartilage that ultimately led to the development of osteoarthritis, especially since you don't have it to the same degree in the opposite knee. A variation on this theme might be the late osteoarthritis that frequently develops in people with a history of congenital joint abnormalities, like a dysplastic or dislocated hip at birth.

"**Obesity is another predisposing factor,** particularly for weight-bearing joints like the hip and knee.

"Whatever the cause, most theories include some mechanical component of 'wear and tear with inadequate repair' that appears to play a much greater role in osteoarthritis than in other arthritic conditions. The irritation produced by wear and tear causes abnormally robust bone growth locally, which is called hypertrophy, and results in bony spurs around osteoarthritic joints."

Harry asked, "Could we have done something to prevent this from happening?"

Can osteoarthritis be prevented?

"That's a question I'm often asked," replied the doctor. "Given the current lack of understanding of the mechanisms involved, the answer for now is probably no, but there is a lot of research going on with the goal of changing that.

"One fascinating approach is to find ways to speed up the cartilage repair process. A group of hormone-like chemicals—called cytokines—secreted locally in joints influences the maintenance of cartilage, suggesting that it may be possible to promote cartilage repair using one or some combination of these chemicals. Although no such treatment is ready for investigation in humans as yet, the concept is clearly promising.

"A more mundane approach," the doctor noted, "might be to reduce the wear-and-tear process by maintaining appropriate body weight and minimizing activities that are thought to damage cartilage. The role of diet beyond appropriate weight maintenance is controversial. For example, vitamin C, once considered to have protective capability, now appears to increase the severity of osteoarthritis of the knees at high doses, that is, more than 500 milligrams daily.

"On the mechanical side, a great deal of research has gone into developing an understanding of the forces that are exerted on the cartilage surfaces in a weight-bearing joint like the hip or knee during walking, running, twisting, carrying, climbing, and other physical activities. Since the actual weight-bearing surface is small—less than a square inch in a knee, for example—this translates into hundreds of pounds per square inch, with peak pressures in the tons with certain kinds of motion. It's no wonder that these surfaces can break down over time.

The doctor added, "A third approach might be to supply the building blocks of cartilage for the body to incorporate without having to synthesize them from scratch. That is the theory behind the use of such agents as glucosamine and chondroitin sulfate, which are biochemicals important in the structure of cartilage and other connective tissue. Although there is little evidence that taking these substances by mouth has any benefit in cartilage maintenance, they do provide symptomatic benefit for some people with osteoarthritis, and they appear to be safe to use. On the other hand, a recently published Italian study suggests that there may actually be some slowing of the progression of osteoarthritis of the knees in people who take glucosamine. Clearly, further study of this issue is needed before we can determine the value of this approach."

Stella then said, "I think I know a few people with osteoarthritis. How common is it?"

How common is osteoarthritis?

"Very common," answered the doctor. "Osteoarthritis affects almost 21 million Americans, mostly over forty-five years of age, and is responsible for 7 million physician visits annually, according to the Arthritis Foundation. Based on that, it would certainly not be unusual for both members of a married couple in their sixties to have significant osteoarthritis. Furthermore, the Arthritis Foundation estimates that almost half of these individuals do not know what type of arthritis they have and, therefore, are not in a position to make informed decisions about treatment."

Harry asked, "Even though we don't know the cause of osteoarthritis, we must have some idea of whether it is inherited. Is it?"

Is osteoarthritis inherited?

The doctor answered, "At least some forms of osteoarthritis appear to have a hereditary component. Heredity is particularly strong in the case of osteoarthritis of the small joints of the hands, which varies in severity from mild to severe and is more frequent in women. Furthermore, congenital deformities of the hip joint—hip dysplasia—tend to run in families, and they often lead to secondary osteoarthritis. Evidence for heredity of common, everyday osteoarthritis of the spine, hips, or knees is not as clear, but these conditions are so common that, short of identifying a gene for this trait, a hereditary pattern would be hard to recognize.

"There's a rare, familial form of generalized osteoarthritis associated with tall stature and a spinal defect called spondyloepiphyseal dysplasia that has been linked to a specific gene mutation. At least three families with this condition have been identified. The point of mentioning this is not to imply that most cases of osteoarthritis have a genetic component, but rather to illustrate that the condition can be inherited in some cases, perhaps in more cases than we know."

Harry and Stella both spoke at once: "What's the cure?"

Can osteoarthritis be cured?

"Just as it's currently not possible to prevent osteoarthritis, it's also not possible to cure it," answered the doctor. "Nevertheless, many avenues of treatment are available. They fall generally into four categories: local medical, systemic medical, surgical, and mechanical." (See chapter 1.)

Stella wanted to know, "Why are women more commonly affected than men?"

Why is osteoarthritis more common in women?

"The short answer is that we don't really know," answered the doctor. "In fact, most forms of arthritis, including osteoarthritis, are more common and tend to be more severe in women. Exceptions to this are the so-called seronegative spondyloarthropathies (see chapter 5), which tend to be more severe in males. Women are especially disproportionately afflicted by osteoarthritis of the fingers. The nodular deformities seen in osteoarthritic fingers are named according to their location: Those of the outermost, or distal interphalangeal, joints are called Heberden's nodes, and those of the middle, or proximal interphalangeal, joints are called Bouchard's nodes. A recently described genetic variant in the FRZB gene is associated with increased risk of osteoarthritis of the hip in women; this variant gene interferes with bone and cartilage development."

Harry then noted, "You hear a lot these days about osteoporosis. What's that? Is it the same thing as osteoarthritis?"

Is there a relationship between osteoarthritis and osteoporosis?

"There's probably not a direct link between osteoarthritis and osteoporosis, although the two conditions frequently occur together," the doctor replied. "In osteoporosis, the amount of calcium in bone is reduced, and people with this condition are more likely to get fractures than they would otherwise. It's possible that the frequency with which the two conditions occur together relates to the facts that both are more common in women and both become more frequent as people get older. Interestingly, the presence of osteoarthritis in the spine may mask the presence of osteoporosis. The test for bone density measures bony resistance to a measured dose of X-rays. If the bone density is low (due to low calcium content of bone, as in osteoporosis), this resistance is decreased and higher-than-normal amounts of X-rays pass through. But low bone density may not be detectable by this method if bone <u>mass</u> is increased due to the bony hypertrophy, or overgrowth, associated with osteoarthritis of the spine. That's why measuring the bone density of the hip rather than the spine is a better way of assessing a person for generalized osteoporosis."

"So where do we go from here?" asked Stella.

How can we treat this disease?

Harry's treatment

"In Harry's case," the doctor began, "the loss of cartilage we see in the hip joint on the X-ray is moderate in degree, and I think that, for the short term at least, the use of medications, exercises, and joint protection might be good enough. Other than osteoarthritis, Harry's health is good, and he has no other conditions that would make the use of anti-inflammatory medications especially risky. Examples of such conditions would include peptic ulcer disease, poor kidney function, any condition that requires the use of anticoagulants, and asthma.

"**Nonsteroidal [not cortisone-like] anti-inflammatory drugs—NSAIDs for short** —are moderately effective relievers of symptoms caused by inflammation, including pain, redness, heat, and swelling. In some people, they produce excellent relief. These drugs work by inhibiting the cyclooxygenase, or COX, group of enzymes, which are responsible for the production of inflammatory chemicals called prostaglandins. Examples of NSAIDs include aspirin, indomethacin, ibuprofen, naproxen, and many others.

"Over the years, the pharmaceutical industry has brought many such drugs to the marketplace, citing improvements such as longer duration of action and/or lower risk of toxicity to justify switching to the latest new drug," the doctor told Harry and Stella. "Some of these drugs have proved so unexpectedly toxic, despite passing FDA scrutiny for initial introduction, that they later had to be removed from the market. Famous examples include benoxyprofen [Oraflex] and zomepirac [Zomax]. Others, such as phenylbutazone [Butazolidin] and oxyphenbutazone [Tandearil] were always known to be toxic and were removed when less dangerous alternatives became available.

"Recently a **new class of NSAIDs, the COX-2 inhibitors**, the prototypes of which are celecoxib, rofecoxib, and valdecoxib, became available. Rofecoxib, which was sold under the brand name Vioxx, had to be withdrawn from the market in September 2004 because a large study showed that it predisposed people to heart attacks. Valdecoxib followed suit in April 2005. There are also some data indicating that celecoxib may have the same problem, though perhaps not as severe. Because they selectively inhibit only cyclooxygenase-2, these drugs should theoretically be less likely to cause gastrointestinal bleeding. **The jury is still out on whether any of the COX-2 inhibitors add sufficient value to warrant their significantly higher cost and greater risk.**"

The doctor recommended that Harry try one of the nonselective NSAIDs. He wrote a prescription for **diclofenac**, 75 mg twice daily with food, and warned Harry to watch for any new symptoms that might appear after starting this drug (or any other NSAID), particularly black, tarry stools that might indicate gastrointestinal bleeding. He recommended that while taking the drug, Harry should have certain blood tests done at about six-month intervals, especially blood counts and serum creatinine levels, to detect evidence of blood loss or impairment of kidney function.

The doctor also discussed with Harry the importance of keeping his body weight down, not carrying excessively heavy objects, and avoiding unnecessary stair climbing. In addition, he suggested that for cardiovascular fitness, Harry should consider swimming three times a week for at least thirty minutes as his exercise of choice, since that activity, while exercising all muscle groups, does not involve weight bearing. He told Harry again how important it was to avoid or limit any activities that produce pain lasting for more than two hours.

Stella's treatment: knee replacement

In Stella's case, because the knee cartilage was almost gone in the lateral compartment of the knee, resulting in pain, inflammation, a "bone-on-bone" situation on X-ray, and marked deformity and instability of the knee, the doctor recommended that she consider surgery. He pointed out that oral medication would be unlikely to provide adequate symptomatic relief, would not lead to cartilage repair, and would require toxic doses to get any benefit at all. Surgical replacement of the knee joint, on the other hand, would relieve pain and stabilize the joint.

The doctor then discussed with Stella the mechanics of replacement:

• She would need to see an orthopedic surgeon subspecializing in adult reconstructive joint surgery. Some surgeons even sub-subspecialize in a particular joint, such as the shoulder, knee, or hip.

• Once the surgeon agreed that total knee replacement (TKR) surgery was indicated, Stella would need a general physical examination to clear her for surgery, making sure that she didn't have any hidden problems (such as partial blockage of the main arteries of the neck or the coronary arteries) that might increase the danger of the procedure. Then the surgeon would schedule a date for the procedure.

• At some point in the process, the surgeon would discuss the various joint-replacement options—cemented vs. uncemented (porous-surface) implants, various replacement materials and their costs vs. expected useful life, and other matters on which she would make a decision.

• The surgeon would also discuss with Stella the expected recovery period and the rehabilitation process she would need after surgery, so that she would have a reasonably good idea of what she was letting herself in for by going through with the surgery.

• When she understood all this, she would be asked to give her informed consent to have the procedure done.

Stella said, "Let's do it." And they did.

Drugs for osteoarthritis

Nonsteroidal anti-inflammatory drugs (NSAIDs)

Earlier, we considered some of the anti-inflammatory drugs available for use in osteoarthritis. But when doctors select and recommend these medications, they have a much larger list from which to choose than the medications we have looked at so far.

The nonselective NSAIDs that to varying degrees inhibit both COX-1 and COX-2 have been introduced over the past three decades, or if we include aspirin, have been around for nearly a century. And if the list is long in the United States, it is even longer in many other countries. Why are there so many drugs that do almost the same thing? Would patients be any worse off if there were only one or two such drugs?

Bringing a new NSAID to market is a time-consuming and costly process, but some new drugs in this category have been helpful to patients and very rewarding to the patent-holding manufacturers because of some designed-in properties. For example, the early NSAIDs, like indomethacin and ibuprofen, are short-acting medications, and it is necessary to take multiple doses daily to maintain benefit. Some newer drugs, like naproxen, sulindac, and diclofenac, were designed to lengthen the duration of benefit, so that they might need to be taken only twice daily. Piroxicam was the prototype of long-acting NSAIDs that could be taken once daily, and nabumetone provided a somewhat safer once-a-day alternative.

NSAID side effects

Although all the nonselective NSAIDs have about the same toxicity profile over populations of users, there appear to be quantitative differences in specific individuals in the degree to which the different drugs produce various side effects. All the drugs are toxic to the liver, the kidneys, the gastrointestinal lining, the bone marrow, the central nervous system, and the inner ear, but many people take them without suffering any of these toxicities, while others have one or more side effects with one drug, but not another. The processes by which currently unknown (perhaps genetic) host factors influence these differences remain to be determined. At present, finding the right drug for the right person remains largely a trial-and-error process.

The nonselective NSAIDs currently available in the United States include the following drugs. Generic names are given in alphabetical order, followed by common brand names in parentheses (see also appendix B):

- acetyl salicylic acid (aspirin, Ascriptin, Bufferin)

- choline magnesium trisalicylate (Trilisate)

- diclofenac (Arthrotec, Cataflam, Solaraze, Voltaren)

- diflunisal (Dolobid)

- etodolac (Lodine)

- fenoprofen (Nalfon)

- flurbiprofen (Ansaid)

- ibuprofen (Advil, Motrin, Nuprin)

- indomethacin (Indocin)

- ketoprofen (Orudis, Oruvail)

- meclofenamate (Meclomen)

- meloxicam (Mobic)

- nabumetone (Relafen)

- naproxen (Aleve, Anaprox, Naprosyn)

- piroxicam (Feldene)

- salsalate (Disalcid, Salflex)

- sulindac (Clinoril)

- tolmetin (Tolectin)

Selective COX-2 inhibitors

As noted above, there is a new subset of the NSAIDs that selectively inhibits COX-2 without inhibiting COX-1. Prostaglandins produced under the influence of COX-1 have a protective effect on the lining of the lower esophagus, the stomach, and the small intestine (duodenum). Therefore, the rationale behind the use of selective COX-2 inhibitors that spare COX-1 is to reduce the likelihood of NSAID-induced ulcers in the gastrointestinal tract. Although this benefit is not absolute, the COX-2 inhibitors seem to be better tolerated than the unselective NSAIDs by people prone to peptic ulcer disease. The trade-off appears to be a somewhat greater risk of coronary artery disease in people taking these medications, especially rofecoxib and valdecoxib, which were withdrawn from the market because of this problem, as previously noted. The only COX-2 inhibitor currently (as of this writing, in October 2005) available in the United States is celecoxib (Celebrex). Furthermore, these drugs are significantly more expensive than their nonselective counterparts. Applications for approval of two additional COX-2 inhibitors (etoricoxib and lumiracoxib) are pending before the FDA as of this writing, but considering the problems with their predecessors, prospects for their release seem dubious.

Other oral medications

Acetaminophen (also spelled acetamenophen, known as paracetamol in the United Kingdom and Europe, and marketed in the United States as Tylenol) is a familiar pain reliever often used in osteoarthritis. This drug does not inhibit COX-1 or COX-2 and is not strongly anti-inflammatory. It does reduce the level of a recently discovered cyclooxygenase designated as COX-3. This enzyme facilitates prostaglandin production in the central nervous system. The effectiveness of acetaminophen in osteoarthritis is, according to most observers, less than that of the more classical NSAIDs, but some people get significant pain relief from it. **In large amounts, acetaminophen is toxic to the liver.**

Glucosamine, often combined with chondroitin sulfate, is another pain reliever widely used in osteoarthritis. These chemicals are components of cartilage, the cushioning, shock-absorbing gristle found in joints, where they are associated with the protein collagen. The rationale behind the use of these agents is that, since cartilage deterioration seems to be the basic lesion in osteoarthritis, replenishing some of cartilage's building blocks might be beneficial. Whether or not that is true, there is evidence that taking glucosamine and chondroitin sulfate provides some pain relief for some individuals. It is thought to be safe, with a few exceptions, to take these preparations, which are not regulated as drugs, but rather as supplements, by the FDA. **People allergic to shellfish should avoid these preparations, because they are extracted from shellfish.**

Injectable drugs

When an osteoarthritic joint, such as a knee, becomes acutely inflamed, it may be beneficial for the physician to inject anti-inflammatory medication directly into the joint. This can provide rapid relief of pain and swelling, lasting for variable periods of time, sometimes up to several months.

A corticosteroid preparation is the most common category of medication for injection into an osteoarthritic joint. These preparations are analogs of hydrocortisone, and several long- and short-acting forms are available. They are usually injected along with a local anesthetic, such as lidocaine, to give more immediate relief than the corticosteroid alone.

Depending on which joint is to be injected, the procedure may be carried out with the patient sitting or lying down. In order to minimize the risk of introducing an infection at the time of injection, the physician cleanses the skin over the joint carefully with an antiseptic, often an iodine-containing solution followed by alcohol. After that, the physician may locally anesthetize the skin with lidocaine, injected through a small needle, or have an assistant "freeze" the skin with ethyl chloride spray. If necessary, joint fluid is removed for laboratory examination at this time. The corticosteroid injection is then administered through a larger-bore needle. The whole procedure should take no more than five or ten minutes and should produce no more than minimal, temporary discomfort.

Hyaluronan, one of the main components of normal joint fluid, is an alternative medication for injection into osteoarthritic knees. This material is viscous and has lubricating properties. Injected into an osteoarthritic knee joint, hyaluronan sometimes produces dramatic symptomatic relief. The usual routine is a series of three injections separated by one-week intervals. Although hyaluronan is expensive, some feel that it is a more physiological approach to osteoarthritis of the knee than corticosteroid injections.

Response to treatment

Harry's left hip

Harry started taking diclofenac according to his doctor's prescription. He also made the suggested modifications to his activities and actually lost five pounds through careful attention to his diet and regular exercise through swimming. He stopped the vitamin C, which he didn't need anyway. His hip pain improved, but it never went away completely. He had no trouble with the medication and was able to continue taking it for many years.

A year or so after Harry first saw the doctor, his right knee swelled up. The doctor thought it might be a result of unconsciously shifting his weight to the right because of the left hip problem. The doctor X-rayed the knee, found that it had minor osteoarthritis, injected the knee with a corticosteroid preparation, and cleared up the problem. Nevertheless, he told Harry that the relief was probably temporary and that the swelling would probably return. At age seventy-five, Harry had a left total hip replacement with a good result.

Stella's right knee

About four months after Stella and Harry saw the doctor for their osteoarthritis evaluations, Stella had a right **total knee replacement**. The orthopedic surgeon recommended that she have an **uncemented porous-surface implant**, which would be secured by ingrowth of bone rather than cement. She required about six weeks of postoperative rehabilitation, including muscle-strengthening exercises, and she made a gradual recovery. The knee was painless, stable, and much improved in appearance. The scar, which was pretty angry looking initially, gradually improved in appearance.

Stella's hands remained gnarled with osteoarthritis, but they didn't hurt, and they functioned pretty well. After the initial appearance of the Heberden's and Bouchard's nodes, which were initially red and painful (but responded to diclofenac and local heat), the inflammation gradually went away, and Stella was able to stop the drugs without recurrence of pain or apparent further progression of the deformities.

And they both lived happily ever after.

Disease at a glance: Osteoarthritis

Who gets it?

- Women more than men, over age forty-five
- Heredity plays a role in hand disease
- Twenty-one million Americans affected

Joint involvement

- May be polyarticular or monoarticular, symmetrical or asymmetrical
- Cartilage thinning
- Spur formation and osteosclerosis (bony hypertrophy)

Laboratory features

- Acute phase reactants are normal
- Rheumatoid factor is negative

Treatment

- General
    - o Adequate rest
    - o Appropriate exercise
    - o Education
- Medications
    - o Aspirin or other NSAID
    - o Local joint injections
- Surgery if appropriate

Chapter 4
Gout

Onset: The pitchfork from hell

When the alarm went off at six in the morning, Elmer struggled to consciousness only to confront a pounding headache. He had been out on the town the night before with some buddies, celebrating the conclusion of a fat contract that would pave the way for his PR agency to add at least six more employees and move to more plush quarters in the high-rent district. Along the way he had imbibed liberal amounts of wine, and he was seriously hung over. Although he knew from previous experience that his current debilitated state would pass, he was pretty miserable at the moment of awakening. But he hadn't seen anything yet!

The woman at his side was still snoring softly. He thought he remembered that her name was Sandy, but the haze that clouded his mind precluded a clear recollection of the frolic that they must have had the night before (or more accurately, in the wee hours of the morning). To say that Elmer swung his legs over the edge of the bed and hopped out would be a gross mischaracterization of the painstakingly careful, lumbering movements that followed, and it was several minutes before he felt capable of standing up. When he did finally attempt to stand, his entire consciousness was suddenly seized and dominated by a sensation that could only be likened to the piercing of the base of his left big toe by a red-hot nail. That pain, completely focused on a minuscule part of his more than ample body, squeezed out all other awareness of his physical condition. His headache was gone. Nothing mattered but the painful left big toe.

Being the macho sort of guy that he was, Elmer didn't scream or collapse. He quickly lifted the left foot off the floor and choked out a "Damn! That hurts." He sat down heavily on the bed and began to examine his foot. Sandy, or whatever her name was, rolled over toward him and slurred out, "Whassamatta, big guy? You don' feel good?" Elmer didn't answer. He was transfixed by the appearance of his foot, which was swollen and had taken on a purplish hue around the base of the big toe. *Figure 1.* He tried gently rubbing the painful area, but quickly thought better of it after setting off further jolts of pain.

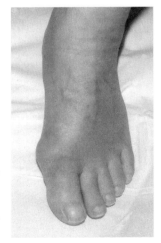

Figure 1: An acute attack of gout in the left big toe. It looks less impressive than it feels (just ask Elmer!).

He became aware that the lethargic voice behind him had become minimally more animated. "You wanna play, honey? Samantha's always ready," the woman said unenthusiastically. Elmer groaned, "Sandy, Samantha, or whatever your name is, you gotta help me. I'm dyin' here." The woman got up and came around the bed. She bent down, took the foot in her hand, and knelt to kiss it. As her lips touched the fevered toe, Elmer finally did scream in pain. "What the hell're you doing? I've got to call my doctor."

Upon hearing the nature of Elmer's problem, the doctor, an internist, suggested that Elmer see a rheumatologist colleague, to which he readily agreed: "Anything to get some relief!"

Initial examination: What did the doctor say?

Samantha drove Elmer to the rheumatologist's office at once and left him there, never to be seen again. Despite bolts of pain, Elmer hobbled into the examining room, unwrapped his throbbing foot (he had not been able to get a shoe on it), and waited. In a few minutes the doctor arrived, gingerly examined the left foot, asked Elmer a few questions, took his temperature, and performed a brief physical examination, focusing on Elmer's skin, particularly around the ears. Then he said, "Well, Elmer, it looks to me like you're having an attack of the gout."

"Well, whaddaya know! My dad had that. I had no idea how bad it hurts. How do I get rid of it?"

"If it is gout, and we need to be sure of that, we can get rid of the acute attack fairly quickly and easily," the doctor replied. "What we probably can't do is cure the underlying problem. But we may be able to prevent further acute attacks, which is almost as good. Once we settle that toe down, we'll have to look at the prevention options and see where we go from here. But before we do any of that, we need to confirm the diagnosis."

"Why do you think this is gout? What else could it be?" asked Elmer.

How did the doctor know the diagnosis?

The doctor explained, "Acute inflammation in a single joint is called monoarticular arthritis, and the list of conditions that cause this is fairly short, with gout leading the list.

"The other main cause of monoarticular arthritis is infection. Although many different infectious agents, including bacteria, funguses, and viruses, can grow in a joint and cause arthritis, generally only bacterial infections tend to cause pain, heat, and swelling of the acuteness and severity that you are experiencing. Infectious agents can get into a joint by two main routes: via the bloodstream or through a local break in the skin. Staphylococcus and streptococcus are the commonest agents infecting joints, but gonococcus, the cause of gonorrhea, is also noted for this."

Elmer's response to this bit of information was "I never had the clap, Doc."

Elmer had no fever, but while the lack of fever increased the odds that his problem was gout rather than infection, the presence or absence of fever is not a reliable differentiator of these two conditions. The doctor noted, "The only way to absolutely rule out a joint infection is by examining and culturing a sample of joint fluid, usually obtained through a needle, since an X-ray would usually still be normal this soon after the onset of symptoms of either gout or infectious arthritis."

Remembering the effects of Samantha's well-intended ministrations to his sore toe, Elmer was not highly enthusiastic about this idea.

The doctor continued, "Occasionally, an injury, especially with a fracture, can mimic acute monoarticular arthritis."

Elmer couldn't remember injuring the foot, but given his condition the night before, he could not rule it out, either.

"A fracture can be ruled out with an X-ray," the doctor went on, "but a sprain does not show up using this method."

Elmer liked the idea of an X-ray better than a needle aspiration of his toe.

"With gout, which is the most likely cause of your problem," the doctor said, "examination of a sample of joint fluid under a microscope is the most reliable way to make the diagnosis. In gout, the inflammation is caused by the formation of monosodium urate crystals in the joint fluid. Sometimes incorrectly referred to as uric acid, monosodium urate—MSU for short—is a breakdown product of cell nuclei. It is not very soluble, and when large amounts of it are present in the body fluids, it can crystallize. MSU crystals are highly inflammatory, and the body tries to get rid of them by mobilizing specialized cells to swallow them up and carry them off. This leads to inflammation. The MSU crystals have a characteristic needlelike appearance. They polarize light, that is, they are birefringent, and they can be identified using a polarizing microscope that employs special filters to determine the direction of polarization of the crystals. The presence of such crystals in the joint fluid is diagnostic of gout."

Elmer listened impatiently to this explanation because it sounded to him as though the doctor was determined to stick a needle into his painful toe. He was right. Elmer was apprehensive, but the doctor reassured him that the pain associated with aspirating the joint would be minimal compared to what he was already experiencing. Although he was dubious about this, Elmer reluctantly acquiesced to the procedure.

Joint aspiration

The doctor called in his nurse. She had Elmer lie down and made small talk with him to calm him down. The doctor cleansed the toe with an antiseptic solution. The nurse handed him a small syringe with a tiny needle filled with a clear fluid. The doctor explained that this was a local anesthetic similar to that used by dentists, which would make the procedure less uncomfortable. He proceeded to inject Elmer's swollen toe with the anesthetic, which produced a burning sensation at the moment of injection. After a short interval, the nurse handed the doctor a larger, empty syringe with a bigger needle. The doctor positioned himself so that Elmer couldn't see exactly what was going on, but Elmer felt a sensation of pressure over the toe, then a sensation of tugging. After a couple of moments, the doctor withdrew the syringe and showed Elmer that he had extracted a small volume of yellowish fluid from the toe. Elmer was surprised at how little the procedure had hurt.

The nurse put some of the fluid into a sterile container for culture and some into a tube for analysis in the lab. The doctor took the nearly empty syringe into another room and looked at a drop of the residual fluid from the syringe through a special microscope under polarized light. He saw needlelike crystals that he determined to be negatively birefringent by rotating the specimen while examining it under polarized light using a special filter (first-order red filter). *Figure 2.*

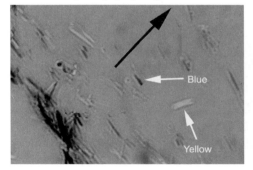

The doctor returned to the examining room and told Elmer that the presence of MSU crystals in his joint fluid confirmed the diagnosis of gout. He added that coexisting infection would not be absolutely ruled out until the culture results were reported a day or two later, but that treatment for acute gout could now be started.

Figure 2: Urate crystals photographed through a polarizing microscope with a first-order red filter. The crystals appear yellow (light colored) when they are oriented parallel to the axis of slow vibration (arrow) and blue (dark) when they are perpendicular to it. This is called negative birefringence, and it is characteristic of urate crystals. Positive birefringence (blue when parallel, yellow when perpendicular to the axis) is characteristic of calcium pyrophosphate dehydrate (CPPD) crystals, found in pseudogout.

Elmer said, "I have a few questions for you, Doc. First off, what tests are you gonna do?"

What tests do I need?

The doctor explained that there were four tests that related to the diagnosis and management of gout:

• **Joint-fluid analysis and culture** would be needed to confirm the diagnosis of gout and rule out infection. The nurse sent the specimens obtained at the time of aspiration to the laboratory for determination of the number and type of inflammatory cells and for culture. Although the lab techs would also look for crystals, this was redundant, since the doctor had already found them.

• **The blood uric acid (urate) level would probably (but not necessarily) be elevated above normal.** The doctor noted that urate levels are often lower during acute attacks than at other times in people with gout. Urate levels provide targets for treatment after the acute attack settles down. In most laboratories, the "normal" range goes up to 7 milligrams per deciliter (mg/dL), but the target for adequate treatment is lower.

• Many doctors determine the **urinary uric acid (urate) excretion rate** by having the patient collect a twenty-four-hour urine specimen and measuring its urate content. The doctor told Elmer that urate is poorly soluble, especially in an acidic environment like urine, and people who excrete large amounts of it are prone to develop stones in the urinary tract. Since some of the older methods for lowering uric acid in the blood do so by increasing its excretion rate, the twenty-four-hour urinary excretion rate may be useful data in selecting a long-term treatment protocol.

• **X-ray of the foot** was useful in Elmer's case because he could not be sure whether the foot had been traumatized, possibly leading to a fracture of one of the small bones of the foot. The X-ray could also show typical changes of infection or of gout, though neither was likely because of timing. Given that this was a first attack, which had begun less than twenty-four hours earlier, the erosions typical of long-standing gout were not likely to be present. In gout, X-rays are more useful if there have been repeated attacks or even chronic arthritis. In a bacterially infected (septic) joint, X-ray changes develop over a period of a few days and would not have been expected in Elmer's case at that time.

The doctor also explained, "Many people with gout have other associated conditions, the most frequent being type 2 diabetes and high lipid levels. Although the time for this evaluation is not necessarily during an acute attack, at some point in the near future, tests for these conditions should be done as a part of your health maintenance program."

"What are you gonna do about my sore toe?" asked Elmer plaintively.

What is the treatment for an acute attack of gout?

The doctor explained that "Depending on the situation, there are several choices for initial treatment of an acute attack of gout. The most rapid and complete resolution of an acute attack can usually be accomplished by using two agents.

• **"ACTH [adrenocorticotropic hormone] by intramuscular injection** gives rapid, complete, but short-duration [about a day] resolution of the acute arthritis of gout. ACTH is a hormone produced by the pituitary gland, a small gland at the base of the brain. Its primary effect is to stimulate the adrenal glands to produce cortisone."

Elmer's response to this was "If that's the case, why not just give prednisone? I took that for poison ivy once, and there are pills for that." The doctor acknowledged the logic of that suggestion, but he pointed out that many physicians who treat gout believe that ACTH has other beneficial effects, not well understood, that make it work better than oral cortisone or prednisone. In many cases, the injection has to be repeated a day later, but generally not beyond that. He went on to tell Elmer about the second medication...

• **"Indomethacin or another fast-acting nonsteroidal anti-inflammatory drug, or NSAID**, such as ibuprofen, diclofenac, and others, has a less potent but more durable suppressive effect on acute inflammation. This medication should be taken at the recommended dosage, beginning at the same time as the first dose of ACTH and continuing for ten days to two weeks."

The doctor also told Elmer,

• **"The classical treatment is colchicine alone**, without ACTH or NSAIDs. Colchicine is a derivative of a naturally occurring chemical found in the autumn crocus. Colchicine tablets, which can be taken at the rate of one per hour until diarrhea occurs, often cool down an acute attack of gout. In many cases, however, this just replaces the problem of gout with the problem of diarrhea, and the use of oral colchicine for acute attacks has, for the most part, joined the ranks of historical treatments that have been replaced by better approaches." The doctor knew that colchicine can also be administered intravenously, however, and its current main use is to treat patients with acute gout who can't take oral medications. This might be the case, for example, during the period immediately after an operation requiring general anesthesia, a common time for a first gout attack in those so inclined.

After ascertaining that Elmer had no history of peptic ulcer disease, asthma, or kidney disease, and that he was taking no medications for anything else, the doctor recommended ACTH, 80 units injected intramuscularly, and indomethacin, 50 milligrams three times daily with meals. He scheduled Elmer for a return visit the next day to evaluate the response and to give another ACTH injection, if necessary. The attack resolved in a few hours, and Elmer felt normal again. Since an acute attack of gout normally lasts only a few days whether it is treated or not, once it has cleared up, the attention should turn to how to prevent another attack.

"I'm all for that," said Elmer. "What are the side effects of all these poisons?"

What are the side effects of treatment for an acute attack of gout?

The doctor explained, "ACTH and cortisone or its analog prednisone suppress the body's ability to fend off infection. If these drugs are administered to someone with an existing, undiagnosed infection, the result can be disastrous, with infection spreading rapidly and destructively. Other acute side effects include fluid retention, flushing, and steroid psychosis. Steroid psychosis is an agitated or euphoric state induced by taking cortisone-like drugs. For reasons nobody understands, the exact symptoms vary in different people. These drugs can also acutely disrupt control of diabetes.

"NSAID side effects include gastric irritation, headache, ringing in the ears [tinnitus], dizziness, asthma, kidney failure, and high blood pressure. Most of these occur more frequently in older individuals. In addition, these drugs interact with certain other medications, such as the blood thinner warfarin, causing them to behave unexpectedly at normal or accustomed doses. Fortunately, you aren't taking any such medications.

"Colchicine causes diarrhea, vomiting, and sometimes suppression of blood-cell production," concluded the doctor.

"Okay, now that we have this thing under control, how do we keep it that way?" asked Elmer.

How do we prevent further attacks of gout?

The doctor answered, "Since attacks of gout occur when MSU crystals form in the joints, lowering the urate concentration in the blood should reduce the likelihood of a gout attack. There are two main methods for accomplishing this: Either increase the rate at which urate is cleared from the bloodstream via the kidneys, or decrease the rate at which urate is produced.

"**Increasing urate clearance was the original strategy for preventing attacks**," the doctor went on. "One method—not very effective—was making the urine less acidic, that is, more alkaline, which increases the solubility of urate in the urine and slightly speeds up clearance of urate from the blood. Over the years, physicians developed several methods for doing this, usually involving the ingestion of large volumes of vile-tasting alkalinizing solutions with multisyllabic names. A better method came with the recognition that probenecid, a drug that was originally developed to decrease the rate at which penicillin was cleared from the body, enhanced the clearance rate of urate from the blood. This was the first really effective method for preventing attacks of gout. Probenecid worked better when the urine was alkaline, so a combination of these two methods worked better than either one alone.

"**The more recent, and clearly more effective, strategy is to decrease the rate at which urate enters the bloodstream.** An early approach to this was to alter the diet so that there would be less precursor substance, or purines, for formation of urate. Although low-purine diets may not be as distasteful as alkalinizing solutions, they are certainly not gourmet delights, and I doubt you would like such a diet," the doctor told Elmer. "But **reduction of urate synthesis is more effectively accomplished by the drug allopurinol and its analogs.** These drugs block one of the enzymes—xanthine oxidase—important in the production of urate from dead cell nuclei. Although blocking this enzyme causes a buildup of the precursors of urate, these are not as insoluble, and they do not fall out of solution and crystallize in the joints. **Thus, urate concentration in the blood falls rapidly when the patient begins taking allopurinol, and this is now the preferred method for prevention of attacks.**

"In gout, MSU crystals build up over time in the tissues and form deposits. When these deposits form in the skin, they are called tophi, and the gout is referred to as tophaceous. *Figure 3.* But similar deposits build up in the joint membranes, and by the time an acute attack occurs, such deposits will have been forming for months to years. If the concentration of urate in the fluids bathing these

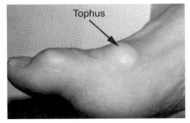

Figure 3: Tophus on the foot of a man with long-standing gout.

surfaces suddenly decreases due to medication, regardless of which strategy is being used to accomplish this, crystal deposits begin to dissolve, and particles composed of MSU crystals may break away from the tissues to which they have become anchored, float free in the joint fluid, and cause inflammation.

"Thus, paradoxical—so-called because urate levels are actually getting lower—gout attacks during the early stages of allopurinol treatment may occur as the urate levels are falling," the doctor warned. "For that reason, during the early months of treatment, it is advisable to take a small dose of colchicine or an NSAID—but generally not both—to prevent attacks until all the urate deposits are dissolved out of the joints and tissues. This may take six to twelve months, after which the anti-inflammatory treatment can usually be discontinued. Allopurinol, however, must be taken permanently, or the buildup of urate crystals and, eventually, the attacks of gout will resume."

"Is there anything that brings on attacks? I was feeling pretty good most of the time till this happened," said Elmer.

What provokes attacks of gout?

The doctor said, "In your case, the attack was almost certainly provoked by the **ingestion of large quantities of alcohol and probably meat** as well. In fact, this relationship, observed over the centuries, is likely responsible for the association of gout with drinking and gluttony in the minds of many people. But plenty of people do the same things you did without having attacks of gout, as indeed you yourself had done previously on many occasions. So there has to be more to it than that.

"**The underlying process—overproduction of urate, probably due to unknown enzyme defects, except for a few cases where the defects are known—must operate for a long time before there is a sufficient accumulation of crystals to cause an attack.**

"**In other cases, attacks of gout may be produced by exposure to lead.** This is called saturnine gout. The people at greatest risk are those involved in the production and consumption of illegal whiskey, or moonshine, because the homemade stills usually contain lead, which leaches its way into the brew. In these cases, it may be a little difficult to tell what is due to lead toxicity and what is due to alcohol, but the lead apparently plays a role, although it is not entirely clear what that role is.

"**Sometimes gout attacks occur in people with cancer as they initiate chemotherapy,**" the doctor said. "The chemotherapeutic drugs cause cancer-cell death on a massive scale, and the dead cell nuclei are broken down by normal pathways, resulting, among other things, in high concentrations of urate as a waste product. Allopurinol is sometimes used to prevent this problem, but since this drug interacts with certain chemotherapeutic agents, caution is advisable.

"**There is evidence that physical trauma can provoke an attack in a joint with extensive urate deposits**, possibly by dislodging some crystals into the joint fluid. Some people believe the big toe is a target joint for gout because of its constant exposure to minor trauma. Proof of this mechanism is limited, but it makes a certain amount of sense," finished the doctor.

"It's hard to believe that my poor toe could hurt so bad and not be damaged in some way. Is there a risk of damage to my joints?" asked Elmer.

Does gout cause crippling disabilities?

The doctor answered, "In your case, what we saw was acute gout, and we made the diagnosis soon after the onset of the first attack. In that setting, there is usually little if any joint destruction, and crippling does not occur.

"However, sometimes gout is not diagnosed or properly treated early, and that's a situation in which a chronic, destructive form of gouty arthritis can develop. This condition resembles chronic, active rheumatoid arthritis in many people. In its intermediate and late stages, chronic gouty arthritis can be diagnosed by examination of joint fluid under polarized light microscopy, and treatment, as I've already described, can halt the progression of the disease, but some damage may remain. This damage may lead to impaired function of the involved joints, which might be a form of crippling. It would be quite rare, however, for gouty arthritis to lead to the need for reconstructive surgery on affected joints."

"I'm glad to hear that," said Elmer. "My old man had this. Are my kids likely to get it?"

Is gout inherited?

The doctor told Elmer, "The genetics of common gout are obscure. According to the National Institute of Arthritis and Musculoskeletal and Skin Diseases, or NIAMS, about 18 percent of those with gout can identify other family members with gout, suggesting the possibility of a hereditary component. For example, you are aware that your father suffered from gout. But many other factors affect the likelihood that a given individual will have gout, including dietary and drinking habits; gender—gout is more likely to occur in males; body weight—obesity is a predisposing factor; and medications being taken, for instance, diuretics, salicylates, niacin, cyclosporine, and levodopa."

"I hate to ask this, but do I need to go on a diet?" asked Elmer.

Does diet help?

Looking hard at Elmer, the doctor told him, "The stereotypical image of the gluttonous, fat, middle-aged male with gout suggests that a more spartan, less excessive lifestyle may reduce the likelihood of gout. Although this image is perhaps a bit overdone, the so-called metabolic syndrome, or syndrome X, is the combination of high blood lipids, hypertension, obesity, and type 2 diabetes. Gout often occurs in this setting.

"As I mentioned, a low-purine diet can help reduce the frequency of attacks in people known to have gout. Foods high in purines [see box], which might cause attacks in those so inclined, include organ meats, certain seafood, game fowl, meat extracts, and dried legumes. If you avoid these foods, you reduce the chance of attacks.

Foods High in Purine Content	
"Organ" meats	**Game fowl**
• Brain	• Goose
• Liver	• Partridge
• Heart	
• Kidneys	**Meat extracts**
• Sweetbreads	• Gravy
	• Broth
Seafood	• Bouillon
• Mackerel	• Consommé
• Herring	
• Shrimp	**Dried legumes**
• Mussels	
• Scallops	
• Anchovies	
• Sardines	
• Roe	

"On the other hand, intake of some foods also reduces the likelihood of attacks, including particularly foods that increase the alkalinity of the urine: fruit juices, especially cherry juice; rice; many vegetables; and dairy products."

"Was that a yes or a no?" asked Elmer. "Never mind. Are there other diseases associated with gout?"

Are other conditions associated with gout?

The rheumatologist answered, "Conditions associated with an increased incidence of gout include illnesses in which there is rapid cell turnover, such as cancer, especially at the onset of chemotherapy, and psoriasis; sarcoidosis, a tuberculosis-like disease of unknown cause; pseudogout, an arthritic condition caused by precipitation of calcium pyrophosphate crystals in joints; obesity; type 2 diabetes; hypertension; lead poisoning; kidney failure; organ transplantation; and high cholesterol. In some cases the mechanisms are fairly well understood, while in others they remain obscure. Although allopurinol can prevent gout, unfortunately it has no effect on most of these conditions associated with gout."

Response to treatment

Within a few hours of receiving ACTH and starting indomethacin, Elmer felt "95 percent better," and by the next day, after receiving the second dose of ACTH, he was completely recovered. The doctor told him, however, that he still had gout, but that taking allopurinol, as noted above, could probably prevent future attacks. Specifically, he recommended that Elmer should follow this regimen:

• Start **allopurinol** at 100 mg daily for seven days, then increase the dose to 200 mg daily for another seven days, then increase the dose to 300 mg daily and continue that dose.

• Start **colchicine** at 0.6 mg twice daily and continue for six months to prevent paradoxical attacks of gout. These are attacks that occur paradoxically as the blood urate level falls rapidly in response to allopurinol.

What lies in store?

It would be nice to be able to say that Elmer could expect to live happily ever after. That would probably be a fair prognosis with respect to his gout, but unfortunately gout seldom exists in a vacuum. Elmer's turbocharged lifestyle carried with it a variety of hazards, going far beyond the health of his joints.

The doctor noted that Elmer probably either had or was at risk for the metabolic syndrome, also called syndrome X. This all-too-common condition is the combination of central (abdominal) obesity, high blood pressure, insulin resistance (including type 2 diabetes), and abnormal blood lipids (predominantly high triglyceride level and low HDL cholesterol). Individuals with metabolic syndrome often have gout along with it. More ominously, metabolic syndrome is also associated with hardening of the arteries (atherosclerosis), heart attacks, and strokes. Although it certainly got Elmer's attention, gout would probably, in the long run, be the least of his problems.

Gout lore

Of all the ills that are known to afflict humankind, very few have accumulated a social lore as rich as that attached to gout. Perhaps the only other disease that comes close in this regard is tuberculosis, with its spas in the mountains, where such people as Hans Castorp went for the cure in Thomas Mann's *The Magic Mountain*. (See chapter 9.)

Gout was not only well known throughout recorded history, having been described by Hippocrates in the fifth century BC, but at times people considered it to be almost a badge of success. In the fifteenth century, Piero de' Medici, who led the Florentine state until his death, was known as Piero il Gottoso, or Piero the Gouty. Piero's father, Cosimo, and son Lorenzo (the family's most famous scion, dubbed the Magnificent) also were afflicted. Interestingly, more recent investigations have cast some doubt on the correctness of the diagnosis of gout in the Medici family, favoring instead ankylosing spondylitis (see chapter 5), an unknown condition at that time.

Cartoons from the eighteenth and nineteenth centuries depict the typical afflicted individual as a well-fed, wealthy, male sufferer, surrounded by his minions and retainers, the aggrieved foot generously wrapped in soft cloths soaked with soothing poultices and supported on a cushion, while Rubenesque female attendants lumber about, responding to his every need. In some old prints and cartoons, many of which have been preserved in the comprehensive collection of the late Dr. Gerald Rodnan, a University of Pittsburgh rheumatologist and connoisseur of gout lore, the devil himself is depicted sticking the painful extremity with a pitchfork.

In the twentieth century, one of the most familiar of the prototype victims of gout was the rotund Jiggs of the *Bringing Up Father* cartoon strip (1913–2000), sitting with his wrapped foot on an ottoman with rays, presumably of pain or heat, emanating from the beleaguered member, being tended to by his sharp-tongued, rather more angular wife, Maggie, and curvaceous daughter, Nora. In those pre-allopurinol days, Jiggs had frequent attacks of the gout, from which he gleaned a great deal of secondary gain.

Disease at a glance: Gout

Who gets it?

- Men more than women
- Associated with type A personality
- Weak heredity component
- 2.1 million Americans affected

Joint involvement

- Typically monoarticular; may be polyarticular
- Most characteristic: big toe
- Acute attacks lasting three to five days

Other features and complications

- Tophi
- Kidney stones
- Neglect leads to chronic, polyarticular arthritis
- May be associated with sarcoidosis, psoriasis, metabolic syndrome

Laboratory features

- Elevated blood uric acid
- Monosodium urate crystals in joint fluid (needlelike, negatively birefringent)
- Often increased uric acid excretion in urine

Treatment

- Acute attack
  - Colchicine or NSAID
  - ACTH or systemic corticosteroid
- Preventive maintenance
  - Allopurinol or other urate-lowering medication
  - Avoidance of dietary indiscretions
  - Adequate fluid intake
  - Education

Chapter 5
Ankylosing Spondylitis and Reactive Arthritis
Onset: Oh, my aching back!

Clyde awoke to the rustling murmur of a soft wind outside his open window, gently disturbing the curtains. It was still dark, but he was having trouble sleeping, as had been the case for the last couple of months, because his back was bothering him. He tried shifting to a new position, but he couldn't get comfortable. As he moved about, he noticed that not only was his back sore, it was stiff as well. He opened his burning eyes and looked at his clock: 3:00 a.m. In about thirty minutes, the alarm would go off, and he would have to get up anyway to study for a histology examination that he was scheduled to take a few hours later. Might as well just get up and be done with it.

At age twenty-two, Clyde was in his second year of medical school, and he couldn't get over how lucky he was. He was the fifth of twelve children. They had all grown up on the family farm in Clarke County, Iowa. Although they always had enough to eat and inexpensive but serviceable clothes to wear, money was perennially tight, and with Dad disabled by arthritis of his back, the kids had to pitch in to get the work done, bring in the crops, and tend to the livestock. When Clyde's older brothers, Wilbur and Clarence, also started complaining of back pain and scaled back their contributions to the effort, Clyde and the younger kids had even more to do. It was hard work, especially at certain times of the year, and the vulnerability of the family fortunes to the bodily infirmities of key players made an indelible impression on young Clyde. He resolved early on to get into a line of work that would make him a little less dependent on his physical strength and robust health.

Hard study and scholarships had gotten him through his undergraduate courses at Iowa State, and from there to the University of Iowa medical school, where he was now toiling his way through the second year of the hardest academic work he had ever known. He was looking forward to getting to the clinical subject matter, especially back pain. Maybe he would be able to figure out the family curse. Old Doc Utterback called it "the rheumatiz," but Clyde thought somehow there might be more to it than that.

Painfully and slowly, he began the daily ritual of getting himself out of bed. There was nothing unusual about the back stiffness, but the pain in his eyes added a new dimension to his discomfort. Within a minute or two, Clyde was able to stand up, but he was unable to straighten completely for about ten minutes, making his way to the bathroom with a hunched-forward posture that made him think of Quasimodo. *Figure 1*. Gradually, as he brushed his teeth, he stretched himself upright. Even deep breathing hurt his back. After a few minutes, when he could position his head so that he could see himself in the mirror, a rheumy, bloodshot pair of eyes stared back at him. "God, I look like a case from *The Crypt of Terror*," Clyde muttered grimly. "I wonder what that's all about."

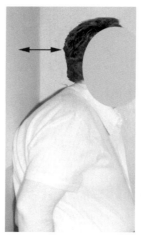

Figure 1: Middle-aged man with moderately advanced ankylosing spondylitis. When he stands with his heels against the wall, he can't touch his head to the wall. Head-to-wall distance, finger-to-floor distance, and chest expansion are classical measurements for following the progress of the disease.

In the end, it was the new problem with his painful, red eyes that scared him. He could live with the back pain, but he didn't relish the thought of trying to practice medicine blind. He went to the student infirmary as soon as he could get himself moving and asked to see the doctor on call.

Initial examination: What did the doctor say?

The doctor running the student health clinic was not much older than Clyde, but he was a nice guy and seemed to know what he was doing. He asked Clyde about his symptoms and appeared interested not only in his eyes but also in his back. It hadn't occurred to Clyde that the two problems might be related. The doctor also seemed interested in the fact that Clyde's father and two of his brothers had similar back problems. He asked Clyde about some symptoms that he hadn't had—rash, mouth ulcers, and, to Clyde's further surprise, drainage from the penis. Then he performed a brief examination, focusing on Clyde's eyes and back.

"Well, Clyde, I'm not entirely sure," the young doctor finally said, "but **I think you have ankylosing spondylitis, and it appears to be complicated by the presence of an inflammatory condition in your eyes called iritis.** *Figure 2*. Ankylosing spondylitis is caused by inflammation in the joints of the spine. It may lead to fusion—ankylosis—of the spinal vertebrae. It's a fairly common form of arthritis, and the susceptibility to it is inherited in a predictable pattern. But I want you to see a rheumatologist to confirm the diagnosis and help us plan the treatment.

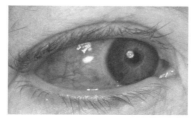

Figure 2: Iritis in a patient with ankylosing spondylitis. Note the prominently dilated blood vessels over the white portion of the eye. This condition, which is also seen in reactive arthritis, is potentially highly damaging to the eye and requires aggressive treatment to avoid visual impairment.

"Iritis, which refers to inflammation in the pigmented layer of the eyes, occasionally occurs in association with ankylosing spondylitis," the doctor explained. "It's a serious condition that needs to be diagnosed and treated without delay in order to relieve pain and protect your vision. I'm going to schedule you for some blood tests and X-rays, but I want you to go see the ophthalmologist right now and let her take a look at your eyes through some special instruments to determine the exact nature of what's going on there."

The ophthalmologist was a pleasant, gray-haired, motherly woman who explained everything she was doing. Clyde thought she was probably a good teacher, whom he would likely encounter again during the course of his studies. She tested his vision, and then she dilated his eyes and looked at them through a scope. She checked the pressure, looking for glaucoma.

Then she said, "Clyde, you do have iritis. I am going to give you a prescription for some cortisone-containing eye drops, and I want you to use them exactly as I prescribe them and for the full course of time, even though your eyes will begin to feel better fairly quickly. It doesn't appear to me that there has been any permanent damage at this point, but it's very good that we are getting started with this treatment early. I need you to come in again in a few days to see how it is going, but if at any time you think your eyes are getting worse, especially if you feel you are losing vision, call me right away."

The doctor's report

A couple of days later, his eyes much improved and feeling good about having passed his histology exam, Clyde went back to the student health clinic to go over the lab and X-ray results with the young doctor. With the doctor was an older man, whom the young doctor introduced, saying, "He is my rheumatology professor, and I have asked him to join us today to give us some advice on what to do."

The rheumatologist shook hands with Clyde and said, "The tests and X-rays confirmed the diagnosis of ankylosing spondylitis. Although you have lost some motion in the lower back, nothing that I see on the films indicates the disease has progressed to the point where you can't get a lot of this motion back with appropriate treatment. Unfortunately, we can't cure ankylosing spondylitis, but we do have pretty good treatment for it. I think we should be able to greatly improve the pain and stiffness and slow down or halt the process of losing mobility in your back."

Using a model, he demonstrated to Clyde the locations of the parts of the pelvis. He showed him how, on the X-rays, the sacroiliac joints of his pelvis were affected. There appeared to be increased bone density along the margins of these joints and some narrowing and irregularity of the joint space. The rheumatologist explained that the pelvis consists of three pairs of bones: the ilia (wings of the pelvis), ischia (the bones you sit on), and the pubes (the small bones in the front of the pelvic girdle). The ilia are connected to the sacrum (lowest vertebrae of the spinal column) through the sacroiliac joints, and the pubes connect through a similar joint (pubic symphysis) in the front of the pelvic girdle. The sacroiliac

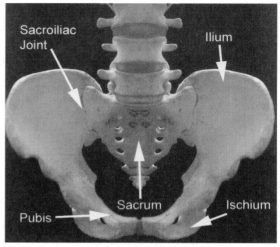

Figure 3: Front view of the pelvis of an anatomical model of the human skeleton. In ankylosing spondylitis, the earliest joints to be affected are the sacroiliac joints, which connect the pelvis to the spine.

joints and the pubic symphysis are fibrous joints with little or no motion under normal circumstances, as opposed to synovial joints like the knees and hips, which move freely. The sacroiliac joints tend to become inflamed in ankylosing spondylitis and generally show the earliest changes that are visible on X-ray in this condition. *Figure 3.*

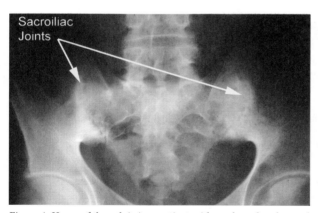

Figure 4: X-ray of the pelvis in a patient with moderately advanced ankylosing spondylitis. The bone immediately surrounding the sacroiliac joints is "sclerotic," that is, densely overgrown and white-appearing on the X-ray, because of stimulation by the presence of inflammation in the joints. The end result of this activity is generally fusion of the sacroiliac joints.

The rheumatologist noted that, although the diagnosis was pretty clear from the symptoms and the sacroiliac joint abnormalities, more X-ray abnormalities would probably be forthcoming, including calcification of the long ligaments at the front and rear of the spine, possibly leading to fusion and the dramatic appearance of the "bamboo spine" that characterizes advanced ankylosing spondylitis. *Figure 4.* He said, "One of our most important jobs in treating ankylosing spondylitis is to avoid having the spine fuse in a forward flexed position. When that happens, it may be impossible for the person to look up high enough to see the horizon." *Figure 5.*

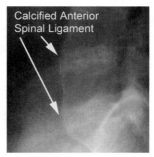

Calcified Anterior
Spinal Ligament

Figure 5: X-ray of a side (lateral) view of the lower (lumbosacral) spine in a patient with ankylosing spondylitis, showing some characteristics of the typical "bamboo" spine. Note the calcium in the anterior spinal ligament, most easily seen in front of the joints between the vertebrae.

The rheumatologist also took note of the fact that one of Clyde's blood tests, the HLA-B27 test, was positive. Clyde's curiosity was piqued.

Clyde's Questions

What is HLA-B27, and what is its relationship to ankylosing spondylitis?

"HLA-B27 is like a blood type, except that it occurs on white blood cells rather than on red cells. About 5 to 8 percent of Caucasians are positive for HLA-B27; it is much rarer in African Americans and almost does not occur at all in pure Africans," answered the young doctor.

"Wow, are you telling me that ankylosing spondylitis occurs in 5 to 8 percent of white people?" asked Clyde incredulously.

Who gets ankylosing spondylitis, and how common is it?

"No, because not all people with HLA-B27 get ankylosing spondylitis," chimed in the rheumatologist. "Ankylosing spondylitis occurs in all degrees of severity, ranging from very mild and almost without symptoms to extremely severe and disabling. About 20 percent of people with HLA-B27 have some evidence of ankylosing spondylitis when you really look for it, but only about one in one hundred develops symptoms severe enough to require treatment."

"What good is a test like that with so many false positives?"

Is there a good test for ankylosing spondylitis?

"I'm glad you asked that question," said the rheumatologist. "A positive HLA-B27 test does not have a high predictive value for the diagnosis, since only 1 percent of such individuals have ankylosing spondylitis severe enough to treat. But since almost all Caucasians with ankylosing spondylitis have a positive HLA-B27 test, a negative result would be strong evidence against the diagnosis. In other words, the HLA-B27 test has a high negative predictive value for the disease, and false negatives are unusual."

"In your case, the clinical evidence in favor of the diagnosis is so strong that the HLA-B27 result has minor confirmatory value in making the diagnosis. If the test result had been negative, however, we might be going back to the drawing board to look for other causes of your symptoms," said the young doctor.

"Don't black people get ankylosing spondylitis?" asked Clyde.

"Ankylosing spondylitis is much less common in blacks than in whites, and when it does occur, the frequency of negative results for HLA-B27 is much higher in blacks than in whites," said the rheumatologist. "The opposite situation exists in certain Native American tribes—Pimas, for example—in whom the frequency of HLA-B27 may be as high as 50 percent and the frequency of ankylosing spondylitis is higher as well. Although in this population there are almost no cases of HLA-B27-negative ankylosing spondylitis, the frequency of false positives is so high that the test is virtually useless. Most ethnic Asian populations have HLA-B27 in about the same proportions as whites, i.e., 5–10 percent in the general population and 95 percent in patients with ankylosing spondylitis. Recent research has focused on the 25 or so subtypes of HLA-B27, which are distributed differently in various ethnic groups. The significance of this finding remains to be determined."

Clyde asked, "Does ankylosing spondylitis affect joints other than those of the spine?"

Does ankylosing spondylitis affect only the spine?

"Not necessarily," the young doctor responded. "Although ankylosing spondylitis always affects the spine, including the lumbar (lower back region), thoracic (chest region), and cervical (neck region) spine, in some people it affects other joints as well, especially the joints of the lower extremities. Hip involvement is fairly common and may be severe, and almost any joint may occasionally become inflamed in this disease. Unlike with rheumatoid arthritis, however, such joint activity is often asymmetrical. While rheumatoid arthritis tends to affect both hips symmetrically, ankylosing spondylitis might affect just one, or it might affect both with greatly differing severity. Nevertheless, like rheumatoid arthritis, this peripheral joint form of ankylosing spondylitis can be very destructive, frequently leading to the need for surgery."

Clyde continued to pursue the topic: "Does ankylosing spondylitis affect only joints?"

Does ankylosing spondylitis affect parts of the body other than joints?

"Ankylosing spondylitis is a systemic disease that may involve various organ systems," continued the rheumatologist, "although arthritis is generally the most prominent component of the disease. As you know from your own experience, Clyde, it can affect the eyes. It can cause painful inflammatory ulcerations in the mouth and nose. It may also be accompanied by a heart murmur due to a leaky aortic valve, known as aortic insufficiency, or an aneurysm—a weakening of the wall—of the aorta, similar to that associated with late stages of syphilis. These aneurysms can rupture with disastrous results. Fortunately, this doesn't occur very often."

"Where does ankylosing spondylitis fit in the grand scheme of the various forms of arthritis?" asked Clyde.

What is the relationship of ankylosing spondylitis to other types of arthritis?

The rheumatologist went on, "HLA-B27 is interesting because, since the association with ankylosing spondylitis became apparent in the mid-1970s, several diseases that had not been previously linked together were found to have a high frequency of HLA-B27 positivity. Prior to that, ankylosing spondylitis was considered to be a form of rheumatoid arthritis, and it was often called rheumatoid spondylitis. Ankylosing spondylitis and related entities are now commonly referred to as the seronegative spondyloarthropathies. The term seronegative means that, as a group, patients with these conditions do not have positive rheumatoid factor tests [see chapter 2]. Besides ankylosing spondylitis, the seronegative spondyloarthropathies include:

- reactive arthritis, which is sometimes called Reiter's syndrome in the United States and Germany and Fiessinger-Leroy syndrome in France;

- psoriatic arthritis with spondylitis;

- enteropathic arthritis with spondylitis; and

- some cases of seronegative rheumatoid arthritis, which have also been called incomplete Reiter's syndrome."

"What is Reiter's syndrome?" asked Clyde.

"Classical **Reiter's syndrome** refers to the triad, or threefold combination, of (a) arthritis, (b) inflammation of the urethra not caused by gonorrhea, that is, nongonococcal urethritis, and (c) inflammation of certain eye structures, such as iritis or uveitis. If any of the three components is missing, the term incomplete Reiter's syndrome would be used. The syndrome sometimes occurs in the setting of a urinary tract infection; a sexually transmitted infection, especially chlamydia; or a diarrheal gastrointestinal infection, as with salmonella or shigella. It may be acute or chronic, and people with HLA-B27 are markedly more susceptible to the chronic form of it than those who lack this genetic marker," explained the rheumatologist.

"I haven't learned about anyone named Reiter in my medical studies," Clyde said. "Who was he?"

Who was Dr. Reiter?

The rheumatologist frowned. "Actually, **the name** *Reiter's syndrome*, which I learned in medical school, **is in the process of being phased out in favor of the term** *reactive arthritis*, which is much more descriptive and avoids the need for an 'incomplete' form of the syndrome. In fact, Reiter wasn't the first to describe reactive arthritis or the triad that bears his name. The new designation recognizes this while tacitly acknowledging recently publicized evidence about Reiter's abominable activities in Germany during the Third Reich.

"Reiter was a committed Nazi who served as the president of the Imperial Health Office—*Reichsgesundheitsamt*, in German—under Hitler. Among other things, he was an advocate of mandatory sterilization and euthanasia as eugenic tools to weed out mental deficiencies and other undesirable traits from the 'master race.' There is widespread agreement that it's inappropriate to reward such unethical behavior with any positive recognition, such as attaching his name to a disease. He was an embarrassment to medicine, and it's wrong to commemorate his name in any way."

Clyde asked, "What happened to him?"

"At the end of World War II, Reiter was interrogated by the Allies, who apparently concluded that they had bigger fish to fry. He was ultimately released without being formally tried and had a long career as a physician and popular lecturer on medical topics, both in Germany and internationally. He died at age eighty-eight at his country estate in Hessen in 1969. His activities on the dark side of medicine became widely known only at the end of the twentieth century, due to the efforts of a dedicated group of American rheumatologists, especially Dr. Dan Wallace, who reviewed and publicized the transcripts of Reiter's postwar interrogations."

"Well, I'm glad I don't have reactive arthritis, although ankylosing spondylitis seems bad enough. What sort of treatment am I looking at?" asked Clyde.

How do we treat ankylosing spondylitis?

The rheumatologist told Clyde that "treatment of ankylosing spondylitis has three components:

- **exercise and physical therapy** to maintain mobility,
- **medications** to control inflammation and pain, and
- **surgery** to deal with damaged joints.

"Of course," said the rheumatologist, "if other organ systems—such as the eyes or the great vessels—are involved, specific treatments for these manifestations need to be considered as well. **There is no cure for ankylosing spondylitis, and it has to be treated as a chronic disease.** Fortunately, with new medications, the outlook is a little brighter for people with the more severe forms of the disease."

Appropriate exercise and physical therapy

"Exercise is extremely important in managing ankylosing spondylitis, and it's the core of the classical treatment program for this disease," the rheumatologist said. "The program has two purposes. The first is preservation of flexibility of the spine. This tends to be a losing battle over time unless the disease goes into a spontaneous remission or is aggressively treated with anti-inflammatory medication. But without an exercise program, loss of mobility is quicker and more complete. The second purpose of physical therapy is to assure that, in the event that mobility is lost, the spine does not fuse in an extreme forward-flexed or twisted position, producing an enormous degree of disability. In the advanced forms of this condition, a person may not be able to raise his head enough to see the horizon, and this is unacceptable to most people."

Anti-inflammatory medications

"Anti-inflammatory medications are the mainstay of drug treatment for ankylosing spondylitis," the rheumatologist explained. "In the early days, when ankylosing spondylitis was considered a form of rheumatoid arthritis, all we had to treat it were large doses of aspirin and the coal-tar derivative drugs phenylbutazone and oxyphenbutazone. In doses that would provide relief of arthritic symptoms, all of these drugs are quite toxic, and treatment was unsatisfactory and dangerous. The Food and Drug Administration eventually banned the latter two drugs from the market because of their unfortunate tendency to wipe out the bone marrow, the place where blood cells are made, causing a potentially fatal side effect called aplastic anemia.

"Indomethacin was a little better, but it was still pretty toxic, especially in elderly people. Corticosteroids would work well for a time but required increasing dosages to maintain effectiveness, and this generated increasing toxicity as well. As time went on, a growing array of anti-inflammatory drugs with different properties and durations of action became available. In the 1980s, **the chemotherapeutic agent methotrexate** became the standard of treatment for rheumatoid arthritis. It's not as effective in ankylosing spondylitis, but it has proved beneficial for some patients."

TNF-alpha inhibitors

"Although the addition of the cyclooxygenase-2, or COX-2, inhibitors [see chapter 2] to the medical arsenal in the late 1990s didn't help much, the advent of the tumor necrosis factor-alpha, or TNF-alpha, inhibitors which immediately followed them may be the long-awaited breakthrough that allows us to treat this disease effectively," the rheumatologist said. "The early results with these drugs are very encouraging, and they do not seem to have insurmountable *short-term* toxicity; only time will tell how well people tolerate them over the long haul."

Surgery

"Many people with ankylosing spondylitis also develop peripheral joint inflammation, especially in the hips, knees, and ankles, and this is typically treated like rheumatoid arthritis," continued the rheumatologist. "Most orthopedic surgical procedures done for patients with ankylosing spondylitis are aimed at peripheral joint disease. Hip and knee replacement surgery and ankle fusions are common procedures performed on patients with ankylosing spondylitis. Surgery on the spine is fraught with hazard and in this disease is best avoided if at all possible. Furthermore, any surgery requiring general anesthesia is difficult when the neck is locked into a bent-forward position. This can make it almost impossible to insert a breathing tube, which must be in place while the patient is anesthetized."

Clyde's treatment

"So, Clyde," said the rheumatologist, "here is what I suggest we do. First, I would like your internist to sign you up for a consultation with Dr. Nelson in Physical Medicine and Rehabilitation. Dr. Nelson will design an exercise program for you and have his therapists teach you what you need to do to remain limber."

The young internist nodded and said, "I'll take care of it."

"In the meantime, I want you to start taking 500 milligrams of **naproxen** twice daily with food. It's a good nonselective anti-inflammatory drug that has to be taken only at twelve-hour intervals. We will give that a trial for a few weeks to see how you tolerate it and how well it works."

Clyde asked, "What are the side effects of naproxen?"

"It has many side effects, the most common of which are upset stomach, ringing of the ears [tinnitus], impairment of kidney function, fluid retention, and hypertension," the young internist said. "It may also cause easy bruising. Prolonged use may lead to peptic ulcer formation and gastrointestinal bleeding, diarrhea, and in some people, impairment of liver function."

"Wow, do you really think it's safe for me to take that stuff?" Clyde asked.

The young internist chuckled. "No medicine is completely safe, but as anti-inflammatory drugs go, naproxen isn't too bad. We'll just have to monitor you closely to make sure we don't get into trouble with it."

"What if it doesn't work?" inquired Clyde.

The rheumatologist answered, "Then we'll have to move on to some of the other drugs."

"Why don't we just start with the safe, effective ones you mentioned, the TNF-alpha inhibitors?" suggested Clyde.

"Eventually, as we learn more about their long-term effects, the treatment protocols may change, and those drugs may become first-line treatments, not only for ankylosing spondylitis, but for many other forms of arthritis as well," said the rheumatologist. "For now, however, if we can get satisfactory control of the disease with drugs that are more familiar, that is probably preferable. So, let's give it a shot, along with the physical therapy, and see what happens."

And that is what they did.

Response to treatment

As initial treatment, Clyde started taking naproxen, 500 mg twice daily, with food. After about ten days, he noticed that the stiffness he experienced in the mornings was somewhat reduced in severity and duration. He also had reduced soreness in his back, though he was certainly not symptom free.

The young internist arranged for him to see the physiatrist for advice and training in an exercise program for ankylosing spondylitis. The physiatrist was a kindly, somewhat elderly man with an interest in medical history, and Clyde enjoyed talking to him. The physiatrist explained that the so-called passive modalities of physical therapy (deep heat, diathermy, ultrasound) might provide some minimal and very temporary relief, enabling Clyde to do the active exercises more effectively. The main benefits, however, were to be obtained from active exercise, particularly stretching exercises. He wrote out a physical therapy prescription and literally put Clyde into the hands of a blonde amazon named Inga. Clyde figured he had better cooperate, since Inga looked as if she could throttle him if she had to. After applying moist heat to his back for a few minutes, Inga showed Clyde how to do the stretching and strengthening exercises for his back that the physiatrist had prescribed and watched him go through a few repetitions. He immediately felt better, and for the first time he began to feel somewhat optimistic about how his treatment was going. Inga smiled and patted him on the head: "You feel better, no?" Clyde nodded, to which she responded, "Good. Go home now and do it."

Complications and first follow-up visit

For the next six weeks, Clyde did his exercises and took his medicine faithfully. Although his back felt better, he was beginning to have a gurgling sensation in the stomach and persistent pains in the abdomen, sometimes burning, other times cramping, which were most unpleasant. His stools first became soft, then watery at times, and finally black and tarry in appearance and consistency. Bowel movements were explosive, accompanied by voluminous gaseous emanations, and required extensive bathroom cleanup. Clyde had seen the 1996 movie *Trainspotting*, and his bathroom at times reminded him of the "worst toilet in Scotland," as depicted in that film. He began to suspect that all might not be well with his medication, and he returned to his internist in the student health clinic.

"Doc, my back feels better, but this medicine is tearing my guts out. Is this what you meant by 'upset stomach'? Isn't there something else that I can take?" asked Clyde.

The internist asked about Clyde's specific symptoms and suggested that he perform a rectal examination in order to test the stool for blood. Clyde warned, "If you stick your finger in there, I can't be responsible for the consequences." The doctor bravely adjusted his glasses, rolled up his sleeves, put on a pair of rubber gloves, and went for it. Somewhat to Clyde's surprise, the procedure went well, and the doctor got his stool sample without incident. He smeared a little on a special paper and applied a drop of developing solution, which almost immediately turned bright blue.

"Your stool test is positive for blood," the doctor told Clyde. "The fact that the stool is black and tarry suggests that the blood is coming from the upper tract, that is, the stomach or upper small intestine; blood from the lower tract, or large intestine, would be red. Like all nonselective nonsteroidal anti-inflammatory drugs, naproxen can cause gastritis or ulcers in the stomach and upper small intestine. It can also cause diarrhea. **You will have to stop the naproxen.** We will need to check you for an ulcer, and if you have one, we will need to treat it. I think that will solve your gastrointestinal problems, but we will probably need to readdress the ankylosing spondylitis," mused the doctor. "**You've experienced what we euphemistically refer to as an adverse drug event, or ADE for short.** Such events are, unfortunately, very common, and they drive up the cost of health care, not to mention causing a lot of misery. There is a lot of interest in finding ways to reduce the frequency of ADEs. But we have a long way to go.

"So, here is what we are going to do:

- First, **stop the naproxen**.

- Second, I will schedule **an endoscopic examination of the esophagus, stomach, and duodenum (upper small intestine) to see if you have an ulcer or significant inflammation in that part of the gastrointestinal tract.**

- Third, I want you to start a new medication called **omeprazole to inhibit acid secretion in the stomach;** this should promote healing of whatever problem is in the upper tract.

- Fourth, I will give you a prescription for **a medication to control the diarrhea;** this medicine is called **loperamide**. You should not need to take it for very long, because stopping the naproxen should resolve the diarrhea relatively quickly if that is the cause."

"Do you think there's a significant possibility that naproxen is not the cause of my diarrhea?" Clyde inquired a little suspiciously.

"Sometimes inflammatory bowel disease occurs in association with ankylosing spondylitis and other seronegative spondyloarthropathies, and it's possible that could be playing a role here," answered the doctor. "We'll see how discontinuing the naproxen affects the diarrhea and proceed accordingly. If the diarrhea doesn't stop, we'll need to do a colonoscopy."

Clyde shuddered. "Sweet Jesus! What next?"

Flare-up and second follow-up visit

The combination of stopping naproxen and starting omeprazole and loperamide was followed quickly by resolution of Clyde's gastrointestinal symptoms. The upper endoscopy (often called EGD, short for esophago-gastro-duodenoscopy) showed only some irritation of the stomach lining, but there was no evidence of an ulcer. The diarrhea cleared almost immediately when the naproxen was stopped. The upper abdominal pain cleared as well. The loperamide and omeprazole were discontinued after a couple of weeks without recurrence of the abdominal pain and diarrhea. But the ankylosing spondylitis symptoms were back with a vengeance.

About a month later, Clyde was in the rheumatologist's office with low back pain and stiffness almost as bad as when he had first consulted the internist. "Well, Doc, what do we do now?"

"Has the diarrhea completely cleared?" asked the rheumatologist.

"Yes, that's not a problem now," responded Clyde. "But this ankylosing spondylitis is cramping my style."

After performing a brief examination, the rheumatologist said, "I agree that the spondylitis is more active again. Are you still doing your exercises?"

"Yes, but they're harder to do now than when I was on medication for the arthritis."

"Okay," said the rheumatologist, "here's what we are going to do next:

- "First, I want you to start **another anti-inflammatory drug,** one that is a specific inhibitor of the enzyme cyclooxygenase 2 (COX-2), called **celecoxib.** This medication is designed to go easy on the gastrointestinal tract. I want you to take one tablet twice daily with food.

- "Second, I want you to start **methotrexate, a chemotherapy drug** that works by inhibiting the body's use of the B vitamin folic acid. This drug also inhibits inflammation by slowing the reproduction of inflammatory cells. Take five tablets each Monday. Methotrexate takes several weeks to work, so don't expect it to produce dramatic benefits overnight, but the celecoxib works a little faster and should help some within a few days. When you come back for your next checkup in eight weeks, we'll see how you are doing and check your blood for toxicity of these drugs.

- In the meantime, I want you to **continue your exercises.**"

Partial improvement and third follow-up visit

Over the next few weeks, Clyde's stiffness improved and his pain lessened. He became able to do his exercises again without much difficulty. He seemed to be tolerating the new medications well. He didn't really feel well, but he was functional and able to go to his classes without great difficulty. The onset of his improvement had been so gradual that he hardly noticed it until he recalled in retrospect how he had felt before. He estimated that he had improved about 50 percent. He still couldn't stand and touch the floor with his knees straight, but instead of missing it by a foot, which had been the case previously, he could now get his fingertips to within six inches of the floor. If he stood with his back to the wall, heels touching the baseboard, he could touch the back of his head to the wall with some difficulty and very little pain.

On his next visit to the rheumatologist, he reported this improvement and asked, "Is it possible to do any better than this? I still feel sort of sick, and I don't have much energy. I always feel like I'm on the brink of disaster, but I keep on rolling along."

The rheumatologist replied, "Until a couple of years ago, there wasn't much more to do for ankylosing spondylitis than what you're now doing. We could get some improvement in most people. But in difficult cases, and especially in situations where people didn't tolerate the medicines well, the outcomes were unsatisfactory, to say the least. Now, however, for people who have tried everything you're on and still aren't doing well, we have some new, powerful biological agents that I've mentioned to you before.

"**These agents block the action of an important inflammatory mediator, tumor necrosis factor-alpha, and they are collectively referred to as TNF-alpha inhibitors or blockers.** TNF-alpha inhibitors have recently been shown to be very useful in treating ankylosing spondylitis. In many patients, their effectiveness is little short of miraculous. The drawbacks are that they're very expensive, must be given by injection, and have unknown long-term side effects. Short-term side effects are not particularly common, but they include headache, cough, pain at the injection site, and increased susceptibility to infection. They have recently been found to unmask latent, unsuspected tuberculosis."

Clyde asked, "How risky are these drugs?"

"Not very risky in the short term, but the answer to your question in the long term is unknown."

"How do we do this?" asked Clyde.

"Although you have no history of tuberculosis or known exposure to it, first we'll get a skin test called a PPD test to make sure that you have no evidence of tuberculosis.

Once we are satisfied that there's no TB lurking in your body, we'll start you on **etanercept** injections, 50 milligrams weekly."

"Okay, Doc. Let's go for it!" said Clyde.

And they did.

Two months later—a miracle

Clyde had a spring in his step. He hadn't felt this good in years. Furthermore, he had passed his semester finals with commendations. He literally danced into his rheumatologist's office.

"Hey, Doc, look what I can do."

He bent forward from the waist and put his knuckles on the floor with no apparent strain.

The doctor commented dryly, "Now you can carry your knuckles close to the ground, just like a normal medical student."

"Aw, Doc, you're just jealous."

And he lived happily ever after, at least so far.

What does the future hold?

For Clyde, the future may be considerably brighter than it is for his brothers Wilbur and Clarence. Both of them have advanced ankylosing spondylitis with bamboo spine changes on X-ray and major areas of fusion of the spine in a forward-flexed position. Poor Clarence can't even watch TV in a normal sitting position. But through careful attention to exercise and medication, Clyde's ankylosing spondylitis does not seem to have produced any permanent anatomical changes in his spine in two years. There are many questions, nevertheless, about how well Clyde will do over the long haul. Will the etanercept, along with his other treatment modalities, continue to hold the disease in check? Will he eventually be able to stop some or all of his medications? Will etanercept produce undesirable long-term side effects that we can only guess at now? And what is the future of celecoxib? We don't know. So far, however, things look good. As with all new treatments, vigilance is the key to long-term safety and success.

Disease at a glance: Ankylosing spondylitis

Who gets it?

- Males get it earlier and more severely than females
- Strong family history
- About 300,000 Americans have ankylosing spondylitis

Joint involvement

- Sacroiliac and intervertebral joints
- Bamboo spine
- Late involvement of peripheral joints

Other features and complications

- Uveitis/iritis (eye inflammation)
- Aortitis and aortic valve disease (similar to syphilitic vascular disease)

Laboratory features

- HLA-B27 positive in more than 90 percent of affected Caucasians
- Acute phase reactants elevated
- Rheumatoid factor negative

Treatment

- General
    - o Adequate rest
    - o Exercise to maintain spinal flexibility
    - o Education
- Medications
    - o Aspirin or other NSAID
    - o Methotrexate and/or other DMARD
    - o TNF-alpha inhibitor
- Surgery if appropriate

Disease at a glance: Reactive arthritis

Who gets it?

- Males more frequently than females

- Strong heredity factor

- May follow urinary tract infection or intestinal infection

Joint involvement

- Tends to be oligoarticular (affecting few joints) and asymmetrical

- May be destructive

Other features and complications

- Iritis/uveitis

- Nongonococcal urethritis

- Psoriasis-like skin rash (keratodermia blenorrhagica)

- Mouth ulcers

Laboratory features

- HLA-B27 usually positive in chronic cases

- Rheumatoid factor negative

- Acute phase reactants often elevated

- Shigella or salmonella may be isolated from stools

- Chlamydia may be found in urine

Treatment

- General

    o Adequate rest

    o Appropriate exercise

    o Education

- Medications for arthritis
    - o Aspirin or other NSAID
    - o Methotrexate and/or other DMARD
    - o TNF-alpha inhibitor
    - o Local joint injections
- Medications for uveitis/iritis
    - o Ocular corticosteroid drops
- Medications for urethritis
    - o Appropriate antibiotic, based on culture
- Surgery if appropriate

Chapter 6
Psoriatic Arthritis
Onset: The heartbreak of psoriasis may be a joint venture

It was two o'clock on a February morning, and Ralph's trio was just finishing their last set. The air in the bar was hazy and heavy with stale cigarette smoke, although only a couple of customers remained. Ralph laid down a few final riffs at the keyboard, scratched his itching scalp, and signaled the group to pack it in. He would be glad to get home that night. The gig had been a bummer. The small "crowd" was dead, the booze was watered, and Ralph, noting that the band now outnumbered the customers, was bone tired and had a headache. Not to mention that for the last few days his hands had felt as if they had molasses circulating through them instead of blood. He'd played almost every slow tune he knew earlier in the evening, but things hadn't loosened up much. Now his hands were starting to ache. Even his hair hurt, he thought.

Arlo, the bass player, caustically observed, "This was a wake, man. If we played any slower, we'd be going backward." Freddy, the drummer, grunted his laconic agreement with that sentiment and began the tedious task of breaking down his equipment for the night. Ralph brushed the dandruff off his collar and responded, "Don't knock it— it pays." Then he headed out through the dirty slush toward his vintage Falcon, which was parked behind the bar. When he got home, he fell into bed and immediately went to sleep.

Later that morning (actually more like noon), Ralph regained consciousness, stumbled into the bathroom, and tried to turn the faucet on the shower, but he found to his surprise that he could not grip it well enough to twist it to the on position. Then he took a closer look at his hands. The thumb and index fingers of the right hand and the index and middle fingers of the left

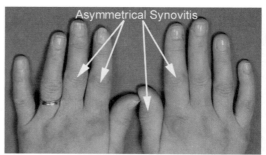

Figure 1: Hands of a female patient with psoriatic arthritis, asymmetrically distributed, like Ralph's arthritis.

hand were swollen up like sausages. *Figure 1*. Both his hands were so stiff that he could hardly move them, and when he tried, his hands felt as though they had been crushed in a car door. This situation was not compatible with the demands of his profession. He had read about the brilliant concert pianist Leon Fleisher, who at the peak of his skills had lost the use of his right hand, devastating his ability to perform. At least

Fleisher always had the use of his left hand and for many years was able to make something of a career out of playing Ravel's *Concerto for Piano (Left Hand)*, but *both* of Ralph's hands were out of commission. Ralph also knew that Fleisher had eventually regained the use of his right hand, and he was determined to seek treatment for his problem immediately. He called his doctor's office and set up a visit for the next day.

Ralph's doctor was a family practice physician. In the doctor's office, Ralph described his problems and his worries about potential disability to the doctor, who asked him a few questions and examined him briefly, then arranged for him to see a rheumatologist whose office was just down the hall. The family physician walked Ralph to the rheumatologist's small suite and introduced him to the doctor, then excused himself and went back to his own busy practice.

After the rheumatologist examined Ralph, among the first questions he asked were how long Ralph's scalp had been bothering him and whether he had any other skin problems. Ralph responded that he had some itchiness in the ears and that he had noted some scaling over the knees and elbows. The rheumatologist then ordered some laboratory tests and X-rays. Before Ralph left the office to get the testing done, the doctor said,"Ralph, the good news is that you don't have what Leon Fleisher had. The bad news is that I think you have psoriasis complicated by one of the common forms of arthritis that can accompany this skin disease. We'll confirm that you have **psoriatic arthritis** by ruling out other forms of arthritis and then get you going on a treatment program. In the meantime, let's start you on an anti-inflammatory medication to try to get you a little more comfortable." He gave Ralph a prescription for **sulindac**, 200 mg twice daily, to be taken with food, and sent him on his way.

The doctor's report

Ralph returned to the rheumatologist's office the following week, having had blood tests and X-rays of his hands and wrists. He was feeling slightly improved on sulindac twice a day, but he was hoping to get a lot more relief than he had achieved so far. The doctor went over the results with him.

"Ralph, the X-rays only showed evidence of soft-tissue swelling around the joints of your swollen fingers. There was no X-ray evidence of damage to these joints. **The only significant abnormality the blood tests showed was evidence of an active inflammatory process; that is, the erythrocyte sedimentation rate was elevated.**"

"What does that mean, Doc?" asked Ralph.

What does an elevated sedimentation rate mean?

"When you have active inflammation in your body, blood proteins are produced that cause red blood cells—erythrocytes—to stick together and settle, or sediment, more rapidly than normal. This is measured in a special narrow glass tube, and the rate at which the cells settle is called the sedimentation rate. An elevated sedimentation rate is a very nonspecific test, and it indicates only that there is inflammation somewhere in your body. It is elevated in many different forms of arthritis. Sometimes successful treatment makes the sedimentation rate return toward normal, and it is used as a rough indicator of the activity of the process."

"Cool. How does that tell you that I have psoriatic arthritis?"

"It doesn't. I can see that you have arthritis, and I don't need a test to recognize that. The sedimentation rate just tells me that your arthritis is active. All your other tests were normal or negative, and in a person with psoriasis, that is consistent with the diagnosis of psoriatic arthritis. **The skin abnormalities I saw at the time I examined you have the typical appearance of psoriasis, and they are located in several of the usual places, that is, the scalp, the ear canals, and over the knees and elbows.**"

"I always thought that psoriasis was a horrible disease with an ugly rash all over the body," Ralph noted. "I didn't even know I had it until you told me. Is it milder in people with psoriatic arthritis?"

Is psoriasis milder in people with psoriatic arthritis?

The doctor responded, "Not necessarily. The skin rash of psoriasis can be of any degree of severity in psoriatic arthritis, and it does not tend to fluctuate in activity with the activity of the arthritis. The relationship between what is going on with the skin and joint activity is complex and not always apparent." He told Ralph that although many people haven't heard of it, psoriatic arthritis is fairly common, and it can take any of five main forms:

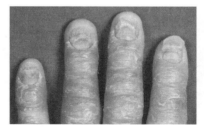

- **One type affects the most distal joints of the fingers**—distal interphalangeal, or DIP, joints—which become swollen and quite painful. *Figure 2.* In this form, the nails usually

Figure 2: Hand of a patient with highly active psoriasis and arthritis attacking the DIP (distal interphalangeal) joints. Note the damage to the fingernails, typical of this form of psoriatic arthritis.

become pitted or pull away irregularly from the underlying nail beds. If the skin involvement is not obvious, this can be easily mistaken for osteoarthritis of the hands.

• **A second type involves mainly the spine** and closely resembles ankylosing spondylitis [described in chapter 5]. This **"psoriatic spondylitis"** is usually accompanied by a positive blood test for the HLA-B27 antigen. Ralph wasn't even tested for B27 because he clearly didn't have spondylitis, based on the clinical picture.

• **The third version, which is what Ralph had, is characterized by involvement of just a few joints—called oligoarticular—usually with an asymmetrical distribution. That is, the same joints are not affected on both sides.** It may or may not be destructive, but if it remains active, the risk of joint destruction is certainly greater.

• **The fourth type looks just like rheumatoid arthritis**, in that it is symmetrical and seropositive; it may represent the co-occurrence of two common diseases—rheumatoid arthritis and psoriasis—rather than a special form of psoriatic arthritis.

• **The fifth type is very destructive and goes by the ominous name of arthritis mutilans."** *Figure 3.*

Ralph asked, "How do you know that this isn't some other kind of arthritis, and that I just happen to have psoriasis, too?"

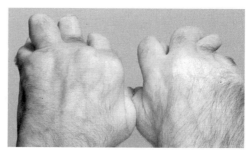

Figure 3: Hands of a patient with the most destructive form of psoriatic arthritis, called arthritis mutilans, for obvious reasons.

How can you tell this is psoriatic arthritis?

"That's a very good question," the doctor acknowledged, "especially since there are at least three other kinds of arthritis that may occur in association with psoriasis.

"The most frequent is probably **rheumatoid arthritis**. Both psoriasis and rheumatoid arthritis are common, and it stands to reason that unless one protects against the other—which does *not* seem to be the case—they would occasionally both be present in the same person on a random basis. But I don't think you have rheumatoid arthritis for a couple of reasons. Your arthritis is asymmetrical, and rheumatoid arthritis is usually symmetrical. Moreover, your rheumatoid factor test is negative. Rheumatoid factor is an antibody that reacts with a normal blood protein called IgG.

About 80 percent of people with rheumatoid arthritis, including those who also have psoriasis, have a positive test for rheumatoid factor; that is, they are seropositive.

"The second form of arthritis associated with psoriasis is **gouty arthritis**," the doctor continued. "Gout is fairly common in people with psoriasis, particularly if the psoriasis is very widely distributed and actively spreading. This probably occurs because in active psoriasis there is rapid cellular turnover in the involved skin, resulting in the generation of a lot of cellular breakdown substances, which include uric acid. Uric acid is not very soluble, and when the concentration in the blood and body fluids, including joint fluid, is high, it tends to crystallize as sodium urate in the joints, causing attacks of gouty arthritis. Your psoriasis is neither widespread nor particularly active, and your uric acid level is normal. Although gout can rarely present as an asymmetrical arthritis affecting a few joints, the most common picture is inflammation of a single joint. If there were any doubt, we could aspirate some fluid from one of your finger joints and look for sodium urate crystals, but this seems so unlikely that I think we can spare you that procedure."

"Thanks," said Ralph, who did not feel that he had been spared much so far.

The doctor went on, "The third is **sarcoid arthritis**. Sarcoidosis is another inflammatory disease that is a little more frequent in people with psoriasis than in the population at large. Although sarcoidosis usually attacks the lungs, once in a while people with this disease have involvement of other organ systems, including the joints. This can take the form of an arthritic condition affecting multiple joints. Since you do not have any other signs of sarcoidosis, for example, abnormalities in the chest X-ray, enlarged lymph nodes, enlarged spleen, enlarged salivary glands, or typical findings of sarcoid arthritis on the joint X-rays, I think we can safely conclude that your arthritis is not due to sarcoidosis."

"Okay, I'm convinced," said Ralph. "What's going to happen to me? Am I going to have to find another line of work?"

Will this disease disable me?

"I hope not," answered the rheumatologist. "In the great majority of people with psoriatic arthritis, the disease can be controlled well enough that they can work pretty much as they did before the onset of disease. As a piano player, however, you have special problems with any condition that affects hand strength and dexterity, and we'll have to see how well you respond to treatment. Fortunately, there are new treatments that are more effective than the previous ones we had, so our success rate in dealing with this disease should be somewhat better than it used to be.

"Nevertheless, in some people psoriatic arthritis can be quite destructive, in much the same manner as rheumatoid arthritis is destructive. If the inflammatory process cannot be controlled, localized damage to cartilage and bone can occur, leading to permanently reduced mobility and to deformity of the involved joints, and even to fusion of the joints.

"At this time, it appears that you have no structural damage to the joints, so in the best–case scenario, if we get an excellent response to treatment, we might expect that your hands could return pretty much to normal."

Ralph was much encouraged by the last statement, and he asked, "What are we waiting for? What do we do next?"

How do we treat this disease?

"Well," said the rheumatologist, "we already have a start on our treatment program in the form of a nonsteroidal anti-inflammatory drug, sulindac. Since you have been taking it in full dosage for about a week, we have a good idea of how well things would go with that drug as the sole treatment. Judging from what you have already told me, I think that sulindac alone isn't going to do the trick."

"I think you're right about that, Doc. Would any other nonst… nonster… What did you call it? Is there another one that would work better?"

"**Sulindac** belongs to the drug class known as nonsteroidal, meaning not cortisone-like, anti-inflammatory drugs. I agree, that's a large mouthful, and **we call such drugs NSAIDs** [pronounced EN-seds] for short. The most familiar NSAID is aspirin. The answer is that there are several such drugs (see pages 16, 30, 32), and it is true that different people react differently to them. When I need an NSAID for myself, sulindac works better for me than any of the others, but some people would say the same for indomethacin, ibuprofen, naproxen, plain aspirin, or any one of a dozen or so alternatives to these drugs. In any given person, it is impossible to say up front which drug would be the best."

"Is Tylenol an NSAID?" Ralph asked.

"Tylenol is one brand name for acetaminophen. It is a pain reliever with only minimal anti-inflammatory activity."

"I can tell you, I'm not very impressed with sulindac," said Ralph, "so what do we do next?"

"The treatment for psoriatic arthritis is similar to that for rheumatoid arthritis. We could try each of the NSAIDs, one after the other, to see which one works best for you," the doctor said. "However, given the minimal response that you got with sulindac, I think it's unlikely, even if there is one that works better for you, that it would produce a completely satisfactory result. Furthermore, it would take several months to give each of the NSAIDs a fair trial, and I don't want to delay more effective treatment that long. **I think we should move to the next step on the treatment ladder, and that would be methotrexate."**

"Man, I've heard of that stuff. Sounds like poison. Are you sure we have to use that?"

"Actually, although methotrexate is a form of chemotherapy, it's pretty safe as drugs for arthritis go. It has also been proven effective in treating psoriasis, but the dosages required to clear up psoriatic skin lesions are much higher than those needed to treat the joints. To be clear about it, I don't think the relatively minimal amount of skin involvement that you have warrants this high-dose treatment at present."

"Easy for you to say, Doc," observed Ralph, not certain that he was happy about having any of his symptoms minimized, "but let's do whatever's necessary to get me going again."

"Okay, then. We'll have you start taking five tablets of methotrexate—a total dose of 12.5 milligrams—each Monday, and you should continue sulindac along with the methotrexate," the doctor told Ralph. "You can expect to see some improvement in your arthritis symptoms in four to six weeks. The improvement may occur so gradually that you will not notice it unless you think back to how you were when you started methotrexate; that is, how you are now. Depending on how you are doing in a couple of months, we have the option of considering additional treatment then, if necessary."

"How often do I need to come back here?" asked Ralph.

"At first, you'll need to come back for follow-up at two-month intervals," answered the doctor. "I'll check your response to the medications and make sure that you're getting adequate improvement. Beyond that, I need to make sure that you're having no side effects from the medications. We'll check your blood count and do some tests of liver and kidney function. If all's well, we can continue the medication as long as it's helping you."

Ralph couldn't think of any more questions, so he took his prescriptions to the pharmacy across the street, got his medications, experienced a moment of shock at the cost of the methotrexate, and went home to start treatment.

Response to treatment

For a couple of weeks after starting methotrexate, Ralph couldn't detect any significant change in his condition, but he stuck with it because he was getting no worse, and there was nothing to suggest the medicine was causing problems for him. He resolved that he would persevere until the first follow-up visit unless things got materially worse. He did, and they didn't.

During this time, he continued to work. Although he didn't feel great, he could still get around the keyboard. He developed an introspective, economical playing style, more like that of the Modern Jazz Quartet's John Lewis than that of his previous model, the flamboyant Oscar Peterson. He found the change to be intellectually challenging, and Arlo, his bass player, got into the spirit of the thing as well, embracing the new fuguelike style. Even the drummer, Freddy, occasionally mustered what passed for a smile in his limited repertoire of facial expressions, but mostly, he just grunted now and then and stared glassily into the great unknown as he brushed his drums.

In his more romantic moments, Ralph began to think of the suffering associated with his arthritis as artistically beneficial. He thought of Chopin, doing his best work as he was slowly being killed by tuberculosis. He was thankful that he wasn't going deaf, as Beethoven did in his later years. The bar patrons really didn't care what the band was playing; they were spiritually benumbed, completely self-absorbed, and focused on the liquid refreshments before them. Ralph thought that they would have been as successfully entertained by the businesslike offerings of Guy Lombardo or Lawrence Welk. As time passed, Ralph increasingly played for hours without even thinking about his arthritis.

First follow-up visit

The two months were up, and Ralph realized that it was time for his first follow-up visit with the rheumatologist. Although he was still having mild swelling and stiffness in several fingers, he had clearly improved. The doctor was impressed with his progress and his success in adapting to the limitations imposed by his condition. But several finger joints were still swollen.

"Doc, I've been slowly improving for the last couple of months, and I'm not sure that I've yet reached the peak of what methotrexate can do for me," opined Ralph. "If my blood tests are okay, I wouldn't mind going on like this awhile longer before we try something new."

"How's your skin doing, Ralph?" inquired the doctor.

"I forgot all about it. I guess it's okay, certainly no worse than before."

"Your blood tests look okay, and there is no evidence of methotrexate toxicity. The only concern I have is that with the arthritis only partially controlled, there's the possibility of joint damage occurring over time."

Alarmed by this, Ralph responded, "I wouldn't want this arthritis to get worse again, especially permanently worse. Considering the amount of improvement I've had, how likely do you think that is?"

"Unfortunately, even though you're clearly a lot better, it's probably fairly likely over time," the doctor replied. "But as you noted, you're still improving, and methotrexate may yet provide adequate control, at least in the short term."

Ralph asked, "So, what's next?"

"I would say our best course of action for now, since your improvement is impressive, is to continue the present treatment and see what happens. In the future, especially if things don't go well, I might recommend that we try one of the new tumor necrosis factor-alpha, or TNF-alpha, inhibitors. There's a growing literature suggesting that these drugs are useful in patients with various forms of inflammatory arthritis, including psoriatic arthritis. Currently, three such drugs are available. The three drugs are etanercept, infliximab, and adalimumab. At this time, only etanercept has been approved by the Food and Drug Administration for use in psoriatic arthritis."

"Tell me more about this. What's TNF-alpha? How well can I expect this to work? Are there any hazards to this treatment?" asked Ralph.

The doctor answered these questions in much the same way that Beulah's doctor had done in discussing her rheumatoid arthritis (see page 19) and Clyde's doctor had done in discussing his ankylosing spondylitis (see page 60): "Although the short-term hazards of using these drugs seem acceptable, we really don't know what problems they may cause after years of use. They do predispose people to infections and these are sometimes serious, but they can usually be successfully treated with antibiotics and temporary withdrawal of the TNF-alpha inhibitor. Nevertheless, the biggest worry is that they may predispose a person to developing certain kinds of malignant tumors, for example, lymphomas, which are much more difficult to treat. Infliximab already seems to be generating lymphomas. We don't know how frequently this may occur, and that will become clearer with time. What we do know is that these drugs often work very well in people with arthritis, and in psoriatic arthritis they may clear the skin lesions as well. One side effect, recently described, is hives, but this doesn't occur very often."

Further course

As the months went by, Ralph's improvement continued. His career took off as well, and over the next few years, at least, he did not have any significant recurrences of his arthritis. He continued to have blood tests several times a year to check for evidence of methotrexate toxicity. On one occasion, he developed a painful mouth ulcer. His doctor had him reduce the dose of methotrexate and added a weekly dose of folic acid, a B vitamin that reduces toxic effects of methotrexate, and the ulcer cleared. He moved, along with Arlo and Freddy, to California, where the weather was more to his liking and where his recording company was based.

And they all lived happily ever after.

Disease at a glance: Psoriatic arthritis

Who gets it?

- People who have had psoriasis for five to ten years (but in a few, the arthritis comes before the rash)

- Males and females equally affected

- Frequent family history

- An estimated 160,000 to 1 million Americans have psoriatic arthritis

Joint involvement

- Five overlapping types:

    o DIP joints with nail changes (10 percent)

    o Rheumatoid arthritis–like distribution (25 percent)

    o Oligoarticular, asymmetrical (80 percent)

    o Spondylitis-like (5 to 20 percent)

    o Mutilans (uncommon)

- Destructive, erosive

- Sausagelike swelling of involved joints

Other features and complications

- Psoriasis, usually with nail changes
- Gout
- Sarcoidosis

Laboratory features

- Elevated acute phase reactants
- Rheumatoid factor usually negative (except for the rheumatoid arthritis–like type)

Treatment

- General
    - o Adequate rest
    - o Appropriate exercise
    - o Education
- Medications for arthritis
    - o Aspirin or other NSAID
    - o Antimalarial drug
    - o Methotrexate and/or other DMARD
    - o TNF-alpha inhibitor
    - o Local joint injections
- Treatment of psoriasis (not discussed in detail here)
    - o Topical medications including medicated shampoo
    - o Methotrexate
    - o UV light (PUVA) therapy
- Surgery if appropriate

Chapter 7
Adult Still's Disease and Juvenile Chronic Polyarthritis

Onset: I've got the fever!

It was summer, but uncharacteristically, Earlene was feeling poorly. She was twenty-eight years old, but she felt as if she were eighty. This was all the more surprising to her in view of the fact that she always kept herself physically fit through eating right, getting plenty of rest, and exercising religiously. She had to because of her job as a guard in the county detention center. She took pride in the fact that under normal circumstances there were no other females and only a few males—either inmates or other guards—whom she could not disable instantaneously with a well-placed kick and a takedown. She was voluptuously good-looking, and several adventurous males had discovered her self-defense skills for themselves. Word had spread, and it was rare that anybody tried anything with her these days.

Today was bad, though. Although this was the fifth time she had felt this way over the past three months, this episode was definitely the worst. Each spell had lasted several days, with the symptoms coming and going once or twice a day. Today, it was hard work just to walk down the hall. She felt alternately hot and cold. She was stiff and her joints were sore. Her hands were diffusely swollen. Earlene noticed there was a subtle, slightly raised, splotchy rash widely scattered over her body. It didn't itch, but when she ran a long, carefully tended fingernail over her skin, she was surprised to see a welt gradually arise in the path her nail had traced. *Figure 1.* Her throat felt sore. She was a mess.

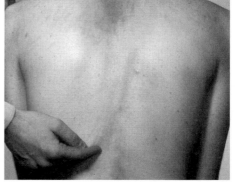

Figure 1: Koebner's phenomenon in a patient with adult-onset Still's disease. Note the broad area of reaction to a light scratch by the physician.

"Hey, sweetie, you don't look so chipper today," yelled 2185906 from his cell. He was leering obscenely at her through the bars, drooling as he retracted his lips to reveal a partial complement of yellow, tobacco-stained teeth. "Why don't you come in here and let me cheer you up?"

"Shut up, jerk. You're not man enough to cheer me up. Besides that, I think I might be coming down with something, and you sure don't want a dose of what I've got."

Earlene headed for the infirmary to see whether she could get some aspirin and was pleased to see that her running pal, Gladys, was the duty nurse. "Man, am I happy to see you, Glad. I'm havin' a bad day, and I feel terrible. I've got a sore throat, and I'm achin' all over. I need something to get me through the rest of this day. What've you got for me?"

"Hey, Earlene, you look like you feel. You'd better sit down here and let me check you over."

Earlene was too sick to argue with her friend. She sat down, and Gladys stuck a thermometer into her mouth. After a few minutes, Gladys removed the thermometer, looked at it, raised her eyebrows, and gave a low whistle. "A hundred and three! Now, that's something." She stuck a tongue blade into Earlene's mouth, turned on a flashlight, and peered over the back of her friend's tongue into her throat. It was red, but otherwise it looked pretty normal.

"Glad, what's this rash look like to you?" asked Earlene.

Gladys looked closely, then shined the light on Earlene's skin and said, "What rash, honey? I don't see anything."

Earlene looked again and was amazed that in the few minutes since she had come into the infirmary, the rash had disappeared.

Gladys took her hand and squeezed it lightly, unintentionally shooting a bolt of pain through Earlene's wrist and forearm. "Yikes, woman, take it easy!" yelped Earlene. "I appreciate the thought, but you don't have to break my hand!"

"Earlene, something's going on here, and we need to find out what. Let's see if one of the young Turks can help us."

She picked up the phone and rang the "doctor" on call. Third- and fourth-year medical students, living and working as externs at the county home for the elderly across the street, took first call at the detention center. Their main job at the home was to pronounce people dead at night so the attending doctors didn't have to come in to do it. If they ran into a problem they couldn't figure out, one of the attending physicians would come over and have a look. It was a flawed system, but chronic personnel shortages at the county facilities made it necessary, and it was a good learning experience for the students.

A half-hour later, a tired-looking young man presented himself in the detention center's infirmary. He perked up a little when he saw Gladys and Earlene, then donned his best professional manner. "What seems to be the trouble?" he asked.

"What's your name, cutie?" asked Gladys playfully.

"Oscar," said the medical student, flushing slightly. He turned to Earlene, who was sitting on an examining table, still in her guard uniform, which she filled impressively. "What's the trouble, ma'am?"

Earlene told him her story, and Oscar listened attentively, making some notes on the chart as she talked. When she finished, he asked her a few questions about her past medical history and family history, especially about any other illness in her family. He asked if she had been around anybody with any infectious illness, to which she replied in the negative. In the review of systems (the part of the medical history in which a series of specific questions pertaining to every system of the body are asked), Oscar asked Earlene if she was sexually active, to which she replied, "Whenever possible." She replied negatively when he asked her about a vaginal discharge.

By this time, Earlene was beginning to feel a little better. When Oscar took her temperature, it had returned to normal. Her throat didn't feel quite as bad, and she was beginning to enjoy the attention.

"Don't you want me to get undressed so you can check me over more thoroughly?" she inquired innocently.

Oscar, now bright red, turned to Gladys and said, "Nurse, prepare the patient for examination," and left the room.

"How old do you think he is, Glad?" asked Earlene as she began to doff her uniform.

"Thinking of 'checking him over more thoroughly,' Earlene? Here, put on this gown, open at the back, and try to control your predatory instincts."

When Oscar returned, Earlene was perched on the end of the examining table, legs crossed, smiling wickedly. Oscar didn't seem to notice. He cleared his throat a couple of times, then began a systematic examination of Earlene, just as he had learned in his physical diagnosis course a couple of years before. Aside from some redness in the back of her throat and some tenderness in the small joints of her hands and wrists, there was not much to find. He confirmed that scratching the skin resulted in the formation, after a few seconds, of a welt along the track of the scratch. He was very careful to ascertain that her spleen was not enlarged, and that there were no enlarged lymph nodes in the neck, armpits, or groin areas, or around the elbows or knees. Throughout the whole procedure, Earlene continued to smile, with her eyes heavy lidded, occasionally moaning softly when Oscar would prod her in various locations, especially the groin. Gladys watched this performance impassively.

"Okay," said Oscar, "I think we're pretty much done here. Why don't you go ahead and get dressed, and then we'll talk about this."

Earlene sat up, allowing the gown to slip off her shoulders. "Let's talk now, Doc," she said.

Gladys immediately stepped over to her, returned the gown to its proper position, and said, "Earlene, behave yourself. You're sick, remember? Oscar, why don't you go next door and write up your findings while I restore some semblance of order?"

With a curious mixture of gratitude and regret, Oscar exited and wrote his notes. When he returned ten minutes later, Earlene was fully clothed and appeared somewhat chastened, although she clearly was feeling much better than she had when Oscar first saw her. Gladys had a grim look on her face.

What was the working diagnosis?

"Earlene," Oscar began, "we need to get a few laboratory tests that will help us narrow down the possibilities, but I think **you may have a rare condition called adult Still's disease. Still's disease is an arthritic condition that usually affects very young children.** The symptoms are swollen painful joints, high fever, a salmon-colored fleeting rash—one that comes and goes quickly, even in a few minutes—sometimes a sore throat, and in many cases a peculiar skin reaction known as Koebner's phenomenon, which I think you have. Let's meet again after we get the tests, and I will go over the results with you and help you get lined up for some treatment."

"Maybe we could do that over dinner," suggested Earlene, "and you could give me my first treatment."

"Earlene, you go to the lab now," ordered Gladys.

The doctor's report

A few days later, Earlene returned to the infirmary as scheduled to meet with Oscar and get her report. Somewhat to her surprise, although Oscar and Gladys were there, also with them was a portly, elderly gentleman whom Oscar introduced as his physician preceptor, a rheumatologist of some local repute who was there to supervise the proceedings.

After the introductions, the rheumatologist said that Oscar's original working diagnosis appeared to be the correct one, and that Earlene, indeed, had adult Still's disease.

"Okay, fellas, you got me," said Earlene. "What's that?"

Earlene's Questions

What is Still's disease, and who was Still?

"Would you like to take that one, Oscar?" asked the rheumatologist.

"I'll give it a shot," ventured Oscar. "I read up on Still's disease after I met Earlene. Sir George F. Still was a British pediatrician whose life spanned the last third of the nineteenth century and the first half of the twentieth. The disease is named after him because he provided the first written description of twenty-two cases of it in his MD thesis in 1896, before he reached the age of thirty. He described what he called 'a chronic joint disease in children.' Ten years later, he became the first chairman of a hospital pediatrics department in England, and in his later years, he was the pediatrician to the royal family, caring for Princesses Elizabeth and Margaret."

Oscar continued, "To expand on what I told you the day we first met, Earlene, Still's disease is an arthritic condition with bouts of fever, often quite high; a fleeting, recurrent, salmon-colored rash; sore throat; and sometimes other symptoms. The fever often has a pattern of one or two peaks daily, up to 103 degrees, with periods of relatively normal temperature in between. The rash tends to be most prominent when the temperature is highest, and it may completely clear in between fever spikes. The arthritis of Still's disease affects multiple joints and may be mild or severe. Although Still referred to the disease as chronic, it isn't always chronic, and it sometimes goes into a complete remission and doesn't recur. When it's chronic, there tends to be destruction of the affected joints unless it's aggressively treated."

"Very good, Oscar," said the rheumatologist. "One of your findings on the initial examination was Koebner's phenomenon. What can you tell us about that?"

What is Koebner's phenomenon, and who was Koebner?

"Heinrich Koebner—usually pronounced KEB-ner by English speakers, originally spelled Köbner—was a German skin doctor, and he practically founded the specialty of dermatology in Breslau, Germany, which is now in Poland and goes by the name of Wroclaw," Oscar related. "He was born about thirty years before Still and died just after the beginning of the twentieth century. In his photos, he looks a little like

Johannes Brahms, the famous, full-bearded German composer, or one of the Smith brothers of cough-drop fame. His most famous accomplishment is that he noticed and described a phenomenon that occurs in psoriasis and certain other diseases, in which mechanical irritation of the skin, such as a scratch, provokes a reaction at the site of the irritation that he called an *'isomorpher Reizeffekt,'* an isomorphic reaction. People liked the term *Koebner's phenomenon* better, and that is what it is called today, in memory of old Heinrich. This reaction to mechanical stimulation is common in Still's disease, but it occurs in many other conditions as well."

"Well done, Oscar," said the rheumatologist.

"Don't get all choked up, Doc," rejoined Earlene. "What else could this be?"

Are there any other diseases this could be?

"I think this is definitely adult-onset Still's disease," said the rheumatologist. "But there are some other diseases that produce fever, rash, and arthritis. When there is a list of diseases that can produce the symptoms a person experiences, physicians call this list the differential diagnosis. Figuring out which item on the differential diagnosis is the cause of the symptoms is a form of medical detective work. Physicians enjoy the intellectual challenge of figuring out the real diagnosis by looking at the differential diagnosis and narrowing the list down. Oscar went through a thought process like this and came up with the right conclusion."

"Wow! I made your day, huh?" suggested Earlene. "I'm glad somebody got their jollies out of this."

"I guess you could say that," Oscar conceded. "Adult-onset Still's disease presents us with a special challenge because there is no lab test that confirms the diagnosis when it is positive. In a way, this is a diagnosis of exclusion: if we can exclude all the other possibilities, then it has to be adult-onset Still's disease, assuming we had all the possibilities on our initial list.

"Certain infections could cause the symptoms you described," Oscar told Earlene. "The ones that come most immediately to mind are gonorrhea and meningococcemia, a bloodstream infection with the germ responsible for bacterial meningitis, but there are others as well. But you didn't have a vaginal discharge, and the blood cultures were sterile. AIDS was ruled out by the lab tests, and I never seriously thought you had it, anyway. Rheumatic fever could also do it, but the throat culture was negative for streptococcus—the cause of rheumatic fever—and the rash wasn't typical. Systemic lupus erythematosus is an autoimmune disease that can produce similar symptoms, but the lab tests for lupus were negative, and the distribution of the rash wasn't confined to sun-exposed areas of skin as in lupus. Occasionally, certain forms of leukemia can also start this way. Again, the lab tests ruled this out. Anyway, you didn't have an enlarged spleen or lymph nodes, and that also ruled out leukemia. The fleeting nature of the symptoms is more suggestive of adult-onset Still's disease than anything else."

"Hey, guys, if this is a childhood form of arthritis, how come I've got it? I'm not a child," Earlene unnecessarily reminded them.

How does Still's disease fit into the spectrum of arthritis?

"Indeed, you're quite obviously not a child," observed the rheumatologist. "But adults can have Still's disease in two different ways. Still's disease can be chronic; it can start in childhood and persist into adulthood, although in many cases, as Oscar has said, it goes into a permanent remission. However, the condition we typically call adult Still's disease has its onset in adulthood, and it is more correctly referred to as adult-*onset* Still's disease. Since the cause is unknown, and the reason for the relationship to childhood is not clear either, we probably shouldn't be too surprised that it can begin in adults. But diseases that begin in unusual ways, especially rare ones, are harder to diagnose because we usually don't think of them in that context. So, Oscar did a good job figuring out a tricky diagnosis.

"In children, Still's disease is one of the four common forms of arthritis, the other three being oligoarticular or pauciarticular (meaning few joints); juvenile chronic arthritis; and polyarticular—adult-form—rheumatoid arthritis presenting in childhood. The latter behaves just like rheumatoid arthritis in adults, and it often persists into adulthood.

"The oligoarticular form of juvenile arthritis involves only a few joints, and these are typically asymmetrically distributed—that is, a finger joint or two on one hand and a wrist on the opposite side, or any other combination of two to four joints," the rheumatologist explained. "This form of arthritis occurs almost exclusively in girls, and it is often accompanied by eye inflammation that can lead to blindness if not recognized and treated aggressively. About 60 percent of these patients eventually go into a permanent remission. Those that don't remit eventually become another group of adults with juvenile-onset arthritis."

Earlene frowned. "Did I hear you say you don't know what causes what I have?"

What is the cause of adult-onset Still's disease?

"The cause of Still's disease, whether it starts in infancy, childhood, or adulthood, is unknown," confirmed the rheumatologist. "This is, in fact, true of most forms of arthritis, unfortunately. Theories range from infection to autoimmunity, but there is little or no support for any of these possible mechanisms. In fact, although adult and juvenile Still's disease look alike clinically except, of course, for the age of the patient, we can't really be certain they are one and the same disease or even that all childhood or all adult cases of Still's disease have the same cause. For practical purposes, we assume they're the same because they act alike, but we really don't know for sure."

Earlene then asked, "Does Still's disease run in families?"

Is there a hereditary component to adult-onset Still's disease?

"That's a very interesting and perceptive question," said the doctor. "Adult-onset Still's disease is so rare that the occurrence of more than one case in a family is almost never observed, so it doesn't run in families, as it were. There is nevertheless a considerable amount of evidence suggesting that juvenile arthritis has a hereditary or genetic component, but the focus of these studies has not for the most part been on Still's disease per se. In Still's disease, genetically determined abnormalities have been described in certain chemical mediators of inflammation, but not all investigators have confirmed these. Most recently, a group of Japanese scientists found evidence of a high-level association of a genetically determined abnormality on a mediator protein called interleukin-18, or IL-18 for short, in people with adult-onset Still's disease. They also found IL-18 to be present in higher than normal concentrations in people with adult-onset Still's disease. If that work holds up to further scrutiny by other labs, it could well be the first direct genetic link in the disease. The short answer, though, is that we don't know for sure as yet."

"Then what are we going to do about it?" queried Earlene.

How is adult-onset Still's disease treated?

"That's another good question," allowed the rheumatologist. "I wish the answers were as good as the question."

"That's not what I was hoping to hear!" exclaimed Earlene.

"The problem is that there really aren't enough cases of adult-onset Still's disease to make good therapeutic trials practical," continued the doctor. "Although there clearly are many points of difference between adult-onset Still's disease and rheumatoid arthritis, we tend to treat them alike. They are both inflammatory diseases of unknown cause, and both target the joints. Both conditions can cause joint damage and its consequent disability, and it is therefore important to bring them under control before they cause too much joint destruction.

"We know from experience that the old 'go low, go slow' approach—that is, start with low doses of medications and escalate only after an 'adequate trial' of the least dangerous and least effective drugs, such as aspirin and its analogs—eventually brings the disease under some semblance of control in many patients, but a lot of mischief can occur while we are slowly getting there. So, I recommend starting with a moderately aggressive medication combination that includes the following medications [see chapter 2 for the details of administration and a discussion of possible side effects]:

- Nonsteroidal anti-inflammatory drug, such as naproxen

- Antimalarial drug, such as hydroxychloroquine

- Antimetabolite, such as methotrexate

- Corticosteroid, such as prednisone

"Prednisone, taken initially in moderately high dosage—20 to 40 milligrams daily—usually brings the fever down in a hurry and gets rid of the rash. But we will start all the drugs at the same time and continue the others, which work more slowly, especially hydroxychloroquine and methotrexate, as we withdraw prednisone during the early phases of treatment. If the disease continues to relapse, we may need to consider using the more potent new biological therapies."

"Won't taking all that stuff at the same time make me sick?" inquired Earlene.

What are the side effects of this treatment?

"It could, but it usually doesn't," replied the doctor. "Our goal here is not to make you sicker, but to get you some relief from this disease that you have come down with.

"Every drug there is has side effects," he continued, "and you might experience one or more of them, especially considering the potency of the medications you're going to take. As I mentioned, **prednisone** works rapidly and is likely to improve the arthritis within a few hours. But this drug has many side effects, and if you continue it at this dose for more than a few days, you'll begin to see evidence of these. It is a strong appetite stimulant, and you will eat more and gain weight rapidly with chronic use of prednisone. The weight gain is associated with a characteristic distribution of body fat to the face and trunk, but not to the limbs. It also causes thinning of the skin and easy bruising, particularly on the arms and legs. In addition, it can cause a form of diabetes—high blood sugar and impaired sugar metabolism—and it can lead to osteoporosis, that is, thinning and softening of bone resulting in fractures and curvature of the spine. It also causes acne. Many people who take this amount of prednisone feel euphoric and energized, even to the point that they have difficulty sleeping at night.

"The onset of action of the other drugs is slower. **Naproxen**, a commonly used non-steroidal anti-inflammatory drug, or NSAID, should begin working within a day, but may not reach full potency for several days or even a couple of weeks. The most common side effect of naproxen is upset stomach, but over time the drug can cause peptic ulcers in the stomach or small intestine. Less frequently, it can cause impaired kidney function, hypertension, damage to the liver, and ringing of the ears with hearing loss. Interestingly, after several decades of use, new data suggest that this drug may be associated with an increase in the frequency of heart attacks. This finding comes on the heels of a number of reports of similar problems with the selective COX-2-inhibiting NSAIDs. It is surprising in view of the fact that naproxen is a nonselective NSAID that inhibits both COX-1 and COX-2 and that the drug has been around so long without any hint of such a problem.

"**Hydroxychloroquine** works considerably more slowly, usually requiring eight to twelve weeks to reach full potency against the arthritis. The most common side effects occur in the gastrointestinal tract and can vary from flatulence to nausea and vomiting. The most treacherous side effects are in the eyes, and these can lead to blindness in the worst-case scenario," the rheumatologist told Earlene. "We have to watch for such problems with regular, annual eye examinations. Hydroxychloroquine can rarely cause many other problems, including skin rash; neuromyopathy, or weakness; cardiomyopathy, that is, enlargement of the heart and heart failure; and a blood disorder in people lacking the enzyme glucose-6-phosphate dehydrogenase, abbreviated as G6PDH.

"**Methotrexate** works by inhibiting the body's ability to use the B vitamin folic acid. Folic acid is needed to form DNA, the most important building block for genes, required for cell reproduction. Since in active inflammation, inflammatory cells must reproduce rapidly, methotrexate inhibits inflammation by slowing this reproductive process. It also has an inhibitory effect on other parts of the body where cells reproduce rapidly, including the bone marrow—where blood cells are formed—and the liver. This is the basis for the main side effects of methotrexate—low red or white cells or platelets in the blood and liver damage. These effects are reversible by simply stopping the drug. Methotrexate also can have other side effects, including nausea and vomiting, menstrual irregularities, and drowsiness. Pregnant women or those trying to get pregnant should not take it. Methotrexate takes several weeks to reach its full effectiveness, but generally by twelve weeks, we can tell how well it is going to work for a specific person, although there is some poorly understood variability in this between individuals." (For additional discussion of these drugs, see chapter 2.)

"You said I shouldn't try to get pregnant while taking these medicines. Why is that?" asked Earlene.

Can I have children while taking these medications?

"Methotrexate reduces fertility," the doctor replied, "**but if a woman should happen to become pregnant while taking it or starts it while already pregnant, continued use of methotrexate often leads to a miscarriage.** Furthermore, because of the way methotrexate works, its presence in the mother's body during the early stages of pregnancy, when fetal organs and systems are forming, could lead to malformations in the developing baby. This phenomenon is called teratogenesis. If the fetus survives, it could lead to a variety of abnormalities. It's best to simply avoid the issue by not getting pregnant while on methotrexate."

"But I can have sex, can't I?" asked Earlene with a worried look on her face.

"By all means. Just don't get pregnant."

"No problem!" exclaimed Earlene with obvious relief.

The doctor then gave Earlene several prescriptions, including naproxen, 375 mg twice daily (with food); hydroxychloroquine, 200 mg twice daily; methotrexate, 12.5 mg once weekly; and prednisone, 30 mg once daily.

Response to treatment

Earlene filled the prescriptions on her way home from work that Friday evening and began taking them the next morning. The first change she noticed was that by late Saturday afternoon she was beginning to feel euphoric. She was full of energy and eager to take on big, unpleasant tasks, like cleaning out the garage and the attic. She felt more like a twenty-eight-year-old ought to feel, in her estimation. In addition, her appetite was voracious. She usually got together with Gladys on Saturday night and shared a pizza for dinner. That evening she consumed (inhaled is more like it) three-quarters of a twelve-slice pepperoni pizza, twice her normal intake.

After Gladys went home, she cleaned up the mess and went to bed, but she couldn't sleep. Her mind was racing, pondering repeatedly all the things she was going to do the next day and throughout the coming week. Finally, she gave up, turned on her lamp, and tried to read. Her taste ran to steamy novels, and she was working on a real barn burner. Alas, it was no good; even the purple, though athletic, prose to which she was so addicted couldn't keep her attention. She called her boyfriend, Fred, but he wasn't at home, or at least wasn't answering his phone. She got up, poured herself a glass of merlot, filled the bathtub with hot water, and slipped in for a relaxing soak. After the bath and the third glass of merlot, she began to feel a little drowsy. Around two o'clock in the morning, she finally fell asleep.

The next day, Earlene's joints were less painful, and she continued to feel as though she were running on jet fuel. Fred was finally home from a short business trip, and he came over to see what was going on. As soon as he walked in the door, she was all over him, and before he knew it they were having passionate sex with Earlene as the aggressor. Fred was surprised, but he was flattered as well. As he regained his composure, he asked her, "What did that doctor do to you? I definitely like it!"

She spoke rapidly. "He's treating me for some kind of arthritis, and he gave me a bunch of medicines to take. They must be miracle drugs. I haven't felt this good in years. I cleaned up this whole place yesterday. The only trouble is that I'm really hungry, and if I keep on eating like this, I'm going to turn into a blimp! All I want to do is eat…and have sex, of course."

Fred's brow furrowed. "Nothing new about that. Let's see what you've got there, sweetie pie."

Earlene showed him her new medications. Fred thought for a moment or two, then said, "The only one of these things I've ever heard of is prednisone. I think that's a form of cortisone. I don't know what all the effects of cortisone are, but I do know that it's a strong drug. Did the doctor tell you anything about side effects?"

Earlene frowned. "I think so, but I was a little distracted at the time, and I am not sure I heard everything he said. I remember that he said one of the drugs might make me blind or give me gas, but I haven't noticed any problem along those lines."

That really made Fred nervous. "I think we ought to go see this guy and find out what's going on," he said.

"Fred, honey, take it easy. He scheduled me back for a one-week follow-up visit. I'm sure that I can last until then. Meantime, let's just enjoy the moment!" she said, smiling wickedly. Fred was always a sucker for that particular line of least resistance.

First follow-up visit and subsequent course

At the end of the week, Fred was really tired, but Earlene was still going strong. At the office, the rheumatologist greeted them cordially.

"How are you feeling, Earlene?" he asked.

Earlene chirped, "My joints have never felt better. My fever is gone, and the rash hasn't come back either. In fact, I feel great!"

Fred chimed in, "But, Doc, she's running me ragged. She eats five times as much as she used to. She's awake day and night. And she's at me all the time, if you get my drift. If you don't do something to calm her down, I'm gonna have to go on those medicines just to keep up with her."

"It sounds like we have a little prednisone-induced euphoria here," mused the doctor.

"We don't have it," exclaimed Fred. "She has it! And what's all this stuff about gas and blindness?"

"Fred, I think we should have a little talk," said the doctor. He then proceeded to repeat the treatment plan he had outlined for Earlene the week before, including the side effects of the drugs, focusing especially on prednisone and hydroxychloroquine. Fred listened attentively and calmed down considerably.

"So, now what?" asked Fred.

"Right now, Earlene's arthritis is being controlled mainly by prednisone and, to a lesser extent, naproxen, since the other drugs haven't had a chance to take effect as yet. But she is beginning to have side effects mainly from the prednisone, so we need to reduce the dose. We would have begun to do that now even in the absence of side effects as long as the disease had settled down, which it clearly has."

The doctor then proceeded to outline a plan for gradual prednisone reduction to a more tolerable dose of 5 mg daily over a one-month period, while continuing the other medications. During this time, Earlene's personality, energy level, and (to Fred's relief) appetites returned to her normal baseline, and over the next twelve months the arthritis and other symptoms of Still's disease remained quiet, apparently controlled by the combination of hydroxychloroquine, naproxen, low-dose prednisone, and methotrexate. Although Earlene had a little increased flatulence, no other side effects were apparent, and she was able to work regularly and resume her previous life.

About a year after the initial episode of illness, Earlene began to notice some swelling and stiffness in the small joints of the hands and the wrists. At first, these symptoms were intermittent, but they became more constant over the next couple of months and began to be accompanied by a lot of pain. She had no fever or rash. The doctor advised her to increase the methotrexate to 15 mg per week, but this really didn't provide much relief.

Additional treatment and future course

At the next visit, the doctor proposed the possibility of adding a new drug to her treatment regimen. "I think we're losing ground with your arthritis, even though we have you on a pretty potent treatment program. There is continued evidence of disease activity, particularly in the joints. Although the rash and fever haven't returned, what we have left looks like chronic rheumatoid arthritis, and that—as we discussed a year ago—is one of the three possible outcomes of adult-onset Still's disease.

"If the arthritis continues to smolder, we're going to see some joint damage, which is likely to result in disability. We may be able to prevent that by using one of the new, biological anti-inflammatory agents I mentioned to you previously. These agents block inflammation directly by interfering with the action of TNF-alpha, a potent chemical produced by inflammatory cells. We now have three such agents, and other promising biological therapies are under investigation," continued the doctor.

He went through much the same discussion with Earlene that Beulah's doctor had pursued when he began treating her with etanercept for rheumatoid arthritis (chapter 2). He pointed out that three TNF-alpha inhibitors were available, and he noted that although all three were effective, none of them had been in use long enough for doctors to have a clear idea what the long-term side effects might be.

Earlene said, "Well, if that's the case, give me the one that's been around the longest. I don't want to take any unnecessary chances."

The doctor said, "For our purposes, there's not much of an advantage to using the oldest drug, which happens to be infliximab, since the difference is only a couple of years, and when we refer to long-term side effects, we are really talking about decades. Just the same, infliximab is a good choice. The main disadvantage of inflix-imab as compared to etanercept and adalimumab is that infliximab has to be given intravenously, while etanercept and adalimumab can be injected under the skin by the patient, like insulin."

So, after making sure that Earlene's tuberculosis skin test was negative, her doctor started her on **infliximab** intravenous therapy, eventually lengthening the time between doses from two to six weeks. Although it took a few weeks, Earlene's response to treatment was excellent.

At this writing, Earlene continues to do well. She and Fred are planning to get married. Gladys is to be the matron of honor. Oscar, the young medical student who had made the initial diagnosis, struck up a friendship with Gladys and Fred and kept in touch with Earlene's progress. Fred has asked him to be the best man, although Earlene knows to an absolute certainty that Fred is indeed the best man (although Gladys has her own ideas about that particular issue). And they all lived happily ever after (except for 2185906, who remains incarcerated).

Disease at a glance: Adult-onset Still's disease

Who gets it?

- Very rare
- Males and females
- Not obviously familial

Joint involvement

- Many joints, episodic activity initially
- If chronic, joint destruction is common, large and small joints, tends to be symmetrical

Other features and complications

- Episodic fever
- Episodic rash
- Koebner's phenomenon
- Sore throat

Laboratory features

- Elevated acute phase reactants
- Negative rheumatoid factor

Treatment

- General
    - o Adequate rest
    - o Appropriate exercise
    - o Education
- Medications
    - o Aspirin or other NSAID
    - o Systemic corticosteroid during acute episodes
    - o Antimalarial drug
    - o Methotrexate and/or other DMARD
    - o TNF-alpha inhibitor
    - o Local joint injections
- Surgery if appropriate

Chapter 8
Systemic Lupus Erythematosus
Onset: A sunburn to remember

Phyllis was twenty-four years old and just starting her new job as an apprentice grave digger for the Municipal Cemetery Association. Although she had a bachelor's degree in biology, she had been unable to find work that took advantage of her hard-won skills and also paid a living wage. She had joined the steelworkers' union, which had a section for grave diggers, and she was ready to go to work. She was a husky young woman who had done construction work during summer breaks from college, and she was looking forward to the outdoor work her new job required. Phyllis had learned to operate a backhoe on her construction job a couple of summers previously, and that experience was going to stand her in very good stead. The training in biology didn't look like it was going to be of much value to her, but you never could tell.

It was a hot, sunny August, and the first week Phyllis was basically occupied with learning her way around the cemetery and working with old Enoch, the senior grave digger, who had been with Municipal for thirty-eight years and kept talking about retiring. Then one day, Enoch got sick—sunstroke, they said—and Phyllis was left to carry the load. It was a bad season for West Nile virus infections, and the grave-digging business was booming. That was okay with Phyllis because now she would get a chance to show her new employers what she was made of.

Because it was hot and nobody else was around, Phyllis shed her shirt and worked in her tank top. She heaved to it with a will and dug more graves in a shorter time than Municipal had ever seen. Her graves were very neat, perfectly rectangular, laid out accurately in the prescribed relationship with the adjacent graves, and exactly six feet deep, just the way the bosses wanted them. By the end of the day, Phyllis was extensively sunburned on her face and much of her upper body, but she felt good. She put her shirt back on and left for home, looking forward to a shower and a cool drink with her boyfriend, Harold.

Phyllis and Harold enjoyed a convivial evening, and when he went home, about 10:00 p.m., she fell into bed and went to sleep immediately. The next morning, however, she did not feel at all well. She was weak and achy, and she felt as if she were coming down with some sort of viral infection. Her hands and wrists were particularly painful, and when she looked at them closely, they appeared to be moderately swollen. When Phyllis looked in the mirror a few minutes later, she saw that there was a scaling rash on her face. When she ran a comb through her hair, more than the normal amount of hair stuck in the comb. She noticed that her mouth was sore, and in the mirror she could see what looked like shallow sores on a white background inside her cheek and on the roof of her mouth. *Figures 1 and 2.*

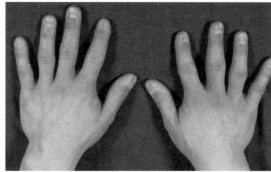

▲ *Figure 1: Hands of a patient with systemic lupus erythematosus and arthritis affecting many of the small joints of the fingers. This arthritis is usually not destructive, although it can rarely cause some deformity.*

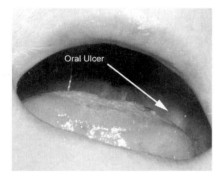

◄ *Figure 2: Mouth ulcers are common in patients with active lupus. They typically are surrounded by a white base. They may or may not be painful.*

"Something's wrong here," Phyllis muttered to herself.

Then she decided to take her temperature because she was feeling alternately hot and cold. It was 103 degrees Fahrenheit. That's when Phyllis decided that a trip to her internist was in order. She called Harold and the Municipal people to let them know what was going on, got herself dressed, hauled herself somewhat painfully into her ancient Yugo, and headed for the internist's office.

When Phyllis arrived, she immediately had to urinate, and, unusually for her, she barely made it to the ladies' room in time. She discharged what seemed to her to be a very large amount of foamy urine. In the process, she noticed that her legs were a bit swollen.

As she returned to the waiting room, she heard the receptionist calling her name, and she was quickly ushered into an examining room. The nurse took her temperature and blood pressure and instructed her to disrobe and put on a gown, open at the back, for examination by the doctor. The nurse also had Phyllis give her a urine sample. Considering how recently Phyllis had emptied her bladder, she was surprised at how much urine she was able to produce.

The doctor entered the room a few moments later and asked Phyllis to describe her problem. After she told him, he inquired about her previous health status, which had always been excellent, and that of her parents and two brothers, also excellent. He then examined her carefully, taking her blood pressure again, looking closely at her rash, the sores in her mouth, her swollen finger joints, and the swelling in her legs, which was severe enough that he could make deep impressions in her flesh with his fingers.

"Phyllis, this might seem like a silly question, but when you get cold, do you notice any color changes in your hands?" he asked.

Surprised, she replied, "My hands have always been sensitive to the cold. When I get cold, my fingers turn dead white, then blue, and as I warm them up, they get very red and feel like they are on fire. How did you know about that?"

"I didn't, and that's why I asked," he said. "You've just given a perfect, textbook description of a condition called Raynaud's phenomenon. Your temperature's gone up to 103.5, and your blood pressure's elevated to 160 over 100."

"What's a normal blood pressure, Doc?" asked Phyllis, who had never really concerned herself with such things.

"For a young person like you, blood pressure shouldn't be higher than 115 over 74, but yours is moderately elevated. Also, the nurse tested your urine sample, and it contained a large amount of protein along with a little blood," answered the doctor.

About that time, Harold showed up. "What's the problem with my girl, Doc?" asked Harold.

Phyllis introduced him to the doctor and said, "Yeah, Doc. Tell us both."

"I think Phyllis may have a condition called systemic lupus erythematosus and that it may be affecting her kidneys. This could be a serious problem, and we need to admit her to the hospital, get a rheumatologist to see her, confirm the diagnosis, and get her on a treatment program."

"What in the world is sys … sys … What did you call it?" they both asked, as with one voice.

What is systemic lupus erythematosus?

The doctor began, "Systemic lupus erythematosus—we call it SLE or lupus for short —is a chronic disease of the immune system. The normal role of the immune system is to recognize large molecules—proteins, polysaccharides, lipids, and nucleic acids— and decide whether they belong in your body or not. When these large molecules interact with the immune system, they are called antigens. The 'decision' as to whether the antigen in question belongs in the body or not depends on whether the immune system recognizes it as native, or 'self'—that is, it belongs there—or foreign, 'not self'—that is, it doesn't belong there. If it's foreign, the immune system attacks it by producing large amounts of antibodies against it. In lupus and other autoimmune diseases, the ability of the immune system to make this distinction is impaired. People affected with lupus make large amounts of autoantibodies that react with their own molecules, whether they are in or on cells or floating free in the circulation. Many of these autoantibodies are harmful and cause the various disease manifestations that we refer to as lupus.

"Depending, at least in part, on the array of autoantibodies produced, the disease has somewhat different characteristics in different people. In SLE, some of these autoantibodies react with components of cell nuclei, which are released into the circulation when cells come to the end of their lifespan and undergo destruction. The most characteristic autoantibodies found in people with SLE are those against DNA, the building blocks of genes, but there are other autoantibodies against cell components as well (e.g., anti-Sm, anti-Ro/SSA, anti-La/SSB, and others). Phyllis, we will be testing you for these and other autoantibodies as a part of your diagnostic workup in the hospital.

"In the blood circulation, these autoantibodies combine with their antigens—the released nuclear components with which they specifically react—and form immune complexes that can move through the circulation and be deposited in various parts of the body, where they cause inflammation. A common location for this deposition of immune complexes is the filtration membranes of the kidneys. When this happens, the filtration process is disrupted, and proteins dissolved in the blood plasma, which are normally too large to pass through the membranes of the kidneys, can now pass through. That causes elevated protein levels in the urine, which you have," the doctor told Phyllis. "Such immune complexes can be deposited elsewhere as well, for instance in the skin, causing a rash; in the joint membranes, causing arthritis; and in other organs of the body, causing a variety of problems."

How did the doctor know the diagnosis?

"For unknown reasons, SLE mostly affects young women. It is much less common for men or older people to come down with SLE, but it certainly can occur. There are eleven criteria that we use to diagnose SLE. These were defined and validated by the American College of Rheumatology back in the 1980s, and they are accepted around the world. If you have an illness in which any four of these are present, the diagnosis is very likely to be SLE, and, Phyllis, you have four. The degree of certainty increases with more than four criteria.

"A first episode of SLE is often provoked by sun exposure, although certain other events can trigger it as well. So, the first clue was the onset of disease after unusual sun exposure and sunburn. That is called photosensitivity, and it is one of the hallmarks of SLE.

"Also, you have arthritis affecting the small joints of the hands. Arthritis is a second criterion for SLE. This type of arthritis tends to be nondeforming, that is, it is unlikely to damage the joints permanently, as rheumatoid arthritis frequently does.

"A third clue is the sores in your mouth. Oral ulcerations, painful or not, are a third criterion for the diagnosis of SLE.

ACR Criteria for the Diagnosis of SLE

- Rash on the cheeks ("butterfly rash")
- Discoid rash (raised, round, red patches)
- Sun sensitivity (photosensitivity)
- Mouth or nose ulcers
- Nondeforming arthritis
- Pleurisy or pericarditis (serositis)
- Renal (kidney) disorder: protein (proteinuria) or cellular casts in the urine
- Neurologic disorder: convulsions or psychosis
- Hematologic disorder: low white cell or platelet count, or hemolytic anemia
- Immunologic disorder: positive LE cell test, anti-double-stranded DNA, anti-Sm, anticardiolipin, or false positive syphilis test
- Positive ANA (antinuclear antibody)

"The fourth clue is elevated protein levels in the urine. This is called proteinuria, and it, too, is a hallmark of SLE.

"In addition, although it is not a formal criterion, the unusual hair loss that you noticed this morning is also suggestive. That is called alopecia, and it is one of the old criteria for SLE. Another suggestive symptom is the Raynaud's phenomenon you described so well.

"Since you have four of the major criteria for diagnosing SLE, the likelihood of the diagnosis being correct is greater than 90 percent, and we haven't even seen what the laboratory will tell us."

At that point, the doctor wrote orders for some blood and urine tests and X-rays and sent Phyllis, along with the faithful Harold, over to the hospital admissions office to arrange for her admission into the hospital and the initial testing. They spent the rest of the day getting Phyllis settled into her room, with a parade of people—staff physicians, doctors-in-training, nurses, technicians, etc.—passing through, asking questions, prodding and poking her, and getting samples of her blood and urine.

Later, Phyllis's internist introduced the rheumatologist to her and Harold. The rheumatologist examined her, talked with them about her condition, outlined a plan for the next few days, and discussed starting her on some treatment. After briefly reviewing the results of the lab that were available by then, the rheumatologist told Phyllis that many of the most important results would be forthcoming over the next couple of days, but that he was pleased to report that her kidney function appeared to be good. Her white blood count was low (a fifth diagnostic criterion for SLE), but she was not anemic. The antinuclear antibody test was strongly positive (a sixth criterion), but the more specific autoantibody test results were not yet available.

Then Phyllis started asking questions.

Phyllis's Questions

What is the cause of SLE, and is it catching?

"The cause of SLE is unknown," replied the rheumatologist. "Genetics appear to play a role, and there is a tendency for SLE to occur in families with other members who have lupus and other autoimmune diseases. But the genetics of SLE are not simple and straightforward. Multiple genes are probably involved, and environmental factors may play a role as well.

"SLE is not known to be contagious, and we think that it isn't. But there have been some intriguing observations that raise questions about this assumption. Family dogs in households where someone has SLE have been reported to have laboratory findings suggestive of SLE. Laboratory personnel who handle blood from people with SLE have a higher-than-expected prevalence of positive tests for antinuclear antibodies. Many viral infections cause temporary elevations of antinuclear antibody levels in people who don't have SLE.

"Could SLE be caused by a virus?" the rheumatologist continued. "It's been suggested, but not proven. With the interest in retroviruses generated by the AIDS epidemic, the possibility of a hard-to-detect virus that disappears into the genetic apparatus of infected cells has certainly received some attention, and the detection of antibody activity that seemed to be directed against the HTLV-1 retrovirus in patients with lupus caused a lot of excitement a few years ago. But none of this has panned out as yet, and all we really have on this point are a number of tantalizing clues, but no definitive proof of anything.

"So, the real answer is that we don't know, but we don't think so."

Phyllis said, "I'm not sure I understood any of that, but do you know how serious my problem is? Can this disease kill me?"

Is this disease going to kill me?

"Well, Phyllis, you're asking me to read the future, and I can't do that," the rheumatologist said. "I can tell you that most people with SLE respond to treatment and live long, productive lives. Some even go into prolonged or permanent remissions, get completely off medications, live to a ripe old age, and die of something else. But some people die of SLE or its complications, including side effects of treatment. Right now, the most critical thing that we need to evaluate is how seriously your kidneys are affected. That is probably the biggest threat to you, at least at the moment. Other onerous complications of lupus, which you don't show any signs of having, include central nervous system symptoms and disorders of the blood coagulation system.

"In order to evaluate the severity of your kidney disease, we will need to obtain a biopsy specimen from one of your kidneys. That'll tell us several things. We'll be able to tell if all parts of the kidneys are involved—diffuse—as opposed to spotty involvement—focal. We will get a look at the nature of the inflammation in the filtration system—the glomeruli—of the kidneys, and see if it's aggressively inflammatory and rapidly progressive (proliferative) as opposed to mildly inflammatory and slowly progressive (membranous) or something in between (membranoproliferative). Using modern technology, we can even see the immune complex deposits and determine where they're located with respect to the filtering, or glomerular, membrane; this gives us additional information about the aggressiveness of the process.

"Finally, we can determine how much of the process is reversible. Once scarring, which can result from unchecked inflammation, occurs, the process is no longer reversible, and this is called glomerulosclerosis. If scarring is widespread, risky treatment has no purpose, and we have to think about dialysis and kidney transplantation.

"At this point, what we have going for us is that you've not been sick very long, and your blood tests suggest that your kidney function is still good—the serum creatinine was normal. Your basic health is good, and we have a little time to figure out where we are with this disease."

"You said we need a kidney biopsy. Do you have to cut me to get that?" asked Phyllis with some trepidation.

How is a kidney biopsy obtained?

"There are two ways to do it," replied the doctor. "The least invasive way is to place a biopsy needle in the kidney through the skin of the upper back under local anesthesia and withdraw a tissue sample through the needle. This often works out very well, and pain associated with this approach tends to be minimal, but there are several things that can go wrong with it. First, because the procedure is normally done blindly, we can miss the kidney entirely and get no tissue or we can get an inadequate sample that does not contain enough kidney filtration units—glomeruli—to allow the analysis we need to conduct. Second, we can't always immediately tell if the kidney, which has many blood vessels, is bleeding after the biopsy specimen is obtained. This can lead to internal bleeding that may not be recognized right away. Open surgery may be necessary to correct either of these problems if they occur.

"The second approach—the one I prefer because it's safer—is to get the specimen through an open surgical procedure, where we can see what we are getting, be sure to obtain a satisfactory specimen, and make certain that there's no bleeding after the procedure is done. The disadvantages of an open biopsy are that general anesthesia is required and the postoperative pain can be significant. The surgical incision also takes longer to heal up than a needle puncture, and it leaves a visible scar.

"Either way, if all goes well, it'll be a few days before we have a result that we can use in determining the treatment that we will pursue, and we'll need to start some treatment now to carry us over until we can formulate a definitive treatment plan."

Phyllis said, "I think I prefer the safer method, even though I might not be able to wear my bikini afterward."

The doctor pointed out that Phyllis's bikini-wearing days were probably over because of the sun sensitivity that goes with SLE and its proven ill effects on her. Harold said, "Amen to that! You need to keep your shirt on when you're outdoors."

Phyllis told him to mind his own business and then turned to the rheumatologist and asked, "How are we going to treat this disease?"

How are we going to treat this disease?

"There will be at least two phases to our treatment: what we do now, and what we do when we have all the information that we'll get over the next week or so. Right now, I am going to start you on prednisone, 60 milligrams daily. That's a moderately high dose. It's not adequate to treat the worst things SLE can do, and it's overkill for mild SLE. But it's a reasonable compromise, given what we know now, and it buys us a little time to get the information we need to develop a more tailored program for you," the doctor told Phyllis. "Over the next week, it's unlikely that you'll have serious side effects, even from that dose of prednisone. But over the long haul, prednisone and the other drugs you're likely to be taking can have significant adverse effects in addition to the beneficial ones, and we need to discuss them before you go home from the hospital.

"We'll need to wait until we see your biopsy and other data before we determine what we're going to do over the next few months," said the doctor.

"One thing I'd like to know now, if you can tell me, is whether this disease affects my ability to have children," said Phyllis. "Harold and I love kids, and we want to have a family someday."

Can I have children?

"At this point, I can't personalize the answer for you because we don't have enough data about you, but I can give you some general information," answered the doctor. "There are three basic issues to consider:

- Will you be able to carry a pregnancy through to term with a healthy baby?

- Would a pregnancy be safe for you?

- What treatment will you need for lupus, and what is its possible effect on the baby?

"SLE may have implications for all of these issues."

Carrying a pregnancy to term with a healthy baby

"SLE per se generally doesn't affect a person's fertility, so getting pregnant would probably be no problem," the rheumatologist told Phyllis. "But there are two conditions that occur in some women with lupus that may make it difficult to carry a pregnancy to successful completion. The more common of these is the presence of autoantibodies that affect the coagulation system. Women with high levels of such antibodies often have miscarriages and have great difficulty carrying pregnancies through to term. One of the tests we're doing on your blood is an assay for anticardiolipin antibodies. Cardiolipin is a lipoprotein antigen similar to that used in the Venereal Disease Research Laboratory [VDRL] test for exposure to syphilis; many people with SLE and certain other diseases have antibodies that react with this antigen. If high levels of such antibodies are present, one of the results may be a tendency to miscarry. They have other implications as well, which we can talk about later, especially if you turn out to have such antibodies. The second condition that may interfere with normal pregnancy is the presence of a particular antinuclear antibody called anti-SSA/Ro. This antibody sometimes cross-reacts with fetal heart tissue, and it can cause a heart rhythm abnormality in the baby that may not be compatible with life."

The safety of a pregnancy for a mother with lupus

"All of us who take care of patients with this disease consider pregnancy as high risk for mothers with SLE because of the observed frequency of flare-ups of the disease during or immediately after pregnancy, even after long periods of relative lupus inactivity," the rheumatologist said. "That doesn't mean a person couldn't try it, but there's a significant risk. It's certainly not advisable to become pregnant while the disease is active; that's asking for trouble."

The effect that treatment might have on the developing fetus

"Many treatments for lupus have the potential of interfering with normal fetal development. This is particularly true of chemotherapy drugs that are used for suppression of the immune system in severe forms of lupus. The risk of fetal death in this setting is considerable, but there's also a risk of producing an abnormal fetus that lives. This is not an attractive set of alternatives.

"But many women with lupus, in whom the disease has responded to treatment and becomes clinically inactive, can have normal pregnancies and healthy children. So pregnancy is not out of the question for you, at least as far as we know now, Phyllis."

"Okay," said Phyllis, "let's go ahead and get the kidney biopsy. I vote for an open biopsy, because I don't want to have to do it again."

"Right," agreed the rheumatologist, "let's do it."

Harold just sat there and looked worried.

Phyllis's blood coagulation tests were normal, and her health was good other than the recent symptoms of SLE. Her anticardiolipin levels were not elevated. Her anti-DNA level, on the other hand, was very elevated, which is consistent with active SLE, and her complement levels were low. Complement is a system of proteins in the blood, similar to the coagulation system, which is activated by inflammatory antigen-antibody complexes. Complement is consumed in the process of generating inflammation, so in SLE, a low complement level usually means that the disease is active. Phyllis's internist consulted a kidney specialist recommended by the rheumatologist to perform the biopsy. The kidney specialist met later with Phyllis and Harold, discussed the biopsy with them, and the biopsy was scheduled for the next day.

The kidney biopsy

Harold sat with Phyllis and held her hand while she waited to be taken to the operating room where the biopsy procedure would be performed. She was nervous about it, but he was the one who was shaking.

"If you ever need a kidney, honey, you can have one of mine," he muttered.

"Oh, stop with that," she admonished him. "This is going to turn out just fine. I've got a feeling about it."

"I hope so," said Harold.

Phyllis was wheeled off to the operating room a few minutes later. Harold came along as far as he was allowed and then went to the family waiting room. Everybody in there looked pretty gloomy, but a cheerful volunteer sat with him and helped the time to pass.

Meanwhile, Phyllis was taken to a brightly lighted room, where a nurse named Gretchen greeted her with a smile and said, "I'm going to just start an IV here, and then we'll get on with it." Gretchen obviously knew what she was doing. She had the IV going almost before Phyllis realized that she had a needle in her arm. Then Gretchen said, "Now I want you to start counting backward from one hundred, and we'll see how far you can get." Phyllis made it to ninety-seven, and everything disappeared.

The next thing Phyllis knew, she was waking up in a new environment. Gradually, she became aware that she was in a large room with several occupied beds and many nurses briskly moving about and checking on their patients. She didn't see Gretchen anywhere, but she noticed that Harold was seated at her bedside.

"What happened," asked Phyllis groggily. "Why didn't they do the biopsy?"

Harold smiled and said, "They did it, and you came through it just fine."

"But nothing hurts," said Phyllis.

The internist, who had just walked in, also smiled and said, "Just wait, Phyllis. You'll be sore soon enough. We'll make sure you get enough pain medication to keep things under control, but the procedure was a success, and we got a nice piece of kidney to examine."

Phyllis went back to sleep, and when she woke up again she was back in her hospital room with the faithful Harold at her side. The doctor was right; she now felt a persistent soreness in the right flank area, where the biopsy had been done. A nurse brought her some pain medication, which she took, and a few minutes later, she fell back to sleep.

The biopsy report and more questions

Phyllis's recovery from the biopsy procedure was uneventful, but the soreness continued for several days, requiring pain medication. The day after the procedure, the rheumatologist came into her room and said that he had looked at the biopsy and discussed it with the pathologist. Although there were a few more studies to perform on the specimens, mainly electron microscopy, he had a preliminary report to give her.

"Phyllis, there is good news and bad news," began the doctor. "The good news is that, as we expected, there is no scarring in the kidney, and it is likely that aggressive treatment will preserve most of your kidney function. The bad news is that the inflammation from lupus is diffuse and involves all the glomeruli that we can see in the specimen. The nature of the inflammation is proliferative rather than membranous, so the process is acute and needs treatment right away. This is called **diffuse proliferative glomerulonephritis. If we leave it untreated, it will probably destroy your kidney function.** So, I recommend that we go ahead with treatment."

"What is the treatment, and how risky is it?" asked Phyllis.

What is the treatment of SLE with diffuse proliferative glomerulonephritis?

"You are already on part of the treatment," said the doctor. "We started you on moderately high-dose prednisone a few days ago, before the biopsy."

"I feel like I'm cured," said Phyllis. "All my aches and pains are gone, except for this biopsy you made me get. Also, my mouth is healing up. How long do I need to take prednisone?"

"I'm glad you're feeling better," said the doctor, "but you're definitely not cured. And you can't continue to take 60 milligrams of prednisone a day indefinitely because of side effects. But for now we will continue it.

"I am going to start you on a medication called cyclophosphamide. We will administer it to you intravenously at monthly intervals. We will give you your first dose later today, while you are still in the hospital. Tomorrow morning, assuming that you tolerate the medication without difficulty, you can be discharged from the hospital, and I will see you in my office for the monthly dose of cyclophosphamide.

"What are the side effects?" asked Phyllis, thinking that she had asked that question before.

How do these medicines work, and what are the side effects of treatment?

Prednisone

"Prednisone has many side effects," the doctor said, "and we are going to have to use it for several months, although we will be reducing it to a lower dose fairly soon.

• **"The most noticeable side effect will be a tendency to gain weight.** Prednisone strongly stimulates the appetite, and almost everybody who has to take it in this dosage gains weight. The distribution of the newly acquired body fat is different from normal obesity. It goes to the trunk and face. The extremities —arms and legs—remain thin. The appearance of someone on prednisone is characteristic, and people familiar with the drug's effects will be able to tell from your appearance that you are taking it. Fortunately, however, this whole process is reversible upon stopping the drug, although it takes some time off prednisone for things to return to normal.

• **"Prednisone reduces a person's resistance to infection, and people taking prednisone in this dosage often get infections, which may be severe.** These infections respond normally to antibiotics, but it is important to recognize them early and get treatment started in a timely manner. Unfortunately, prednisone also masks some of the signs of infection that we will be watching for—for example, fever—so this is not as easy as it sounds.

• **"Prednisone causes osteoporosis, which is reduced bone strength due to low calcium content.** This makes bones soft and increases the likelihood of fractures. We can somewhat reduce this effect of prednisone by having you take supplemental calcium and vitamin D, but we will need to watch your bone density to make sure that we are not getting into trouble as you continue to take prednisone.

• **"Prednisone can cause hypertension, diabetes, acne, thinning of the skin, bruising of the skin, and other problems as well."**

Cyclophosphamide

"**Cyclophosphamide is a chemotherapy drug belonging to the class referred to as alkylating agents.** It is chemically similar to nitrogen mustard, so called because of its resemblance to the mustard gas used in World War I. Cyclophosphamide works by binding to DNA in rapidly dividing cells and killing these cells. In active SLE, the most rapidly dividing cells are the immune cells producing autoantibodies that cause the disease, as well as the inflammatory cells themselves. The goal of using this drug is to wipe out the populations of antibody-producing cells without doing permanent harm to the rest of the immune system or the other cells of the body. Most of the side effects of cyclophosphamide are the result of its tendency to attack other dividing cells at the same time it is doing what we want.

"Because cyclophosphamide is excreted in the urine, the urinary bladder is exposed to it until the bladder empties. The drug can have two very bad effects on the bladder:

• "Cyclophosphamide can irritate the bladder wall and cause hemorrhaging. This can be very severe, and a person can actually bleed to death from cyclophosphamide-induced bladder hemorrhage. So, if you see any sign of blood in the urine, that is a potential emergency, and we need to address it immediately.

• "Irritation of the bladder wall can, over time, lead to cancer of the bladder. This can be treated, but the treatment generally calls for removal of the urinary bladder. If you were to take cyclophosphamide by mouth, your bladder would be exposed to it all the time you're taking the drug. By giving it in monthly intravenous doses, we can minimize the exposure time of the bladder to the drug. Furthermore, we administer a drug called mesna along with the cyclophosphamide to protect the bladder wall. Nonetheless, we must be vigilant about both of these adverse effects of cyclophosphamide, so that if they occur, we can treat them as early as possible.

"Although cancer of the bladder is the most frequent type of cancer that cyclophosphamide causes, it can also cause other forms of cancer, especially lymphoma and leukemia, and we need to watch for these as well.

• "Cyclophosphamide, like many forms of chemotherapy, also can cause nausea and vomiting. To prevent this, with each dose of cyclophosphamide and mesna we include a dose of ondansetron, a strong antinausea medication. This usually completely prevents nausea and vomiting.

• "Cyclophosphamide is also prone to cause hair loss. With the dosage of cyclophosphamide that we use in treating SLE, we sometimes see it but certainly not always. This hair loss, though it can lead to total baldness, is completely reversible, and when the drug is stopped after the course of treatment is finished, the hair grows back normally. Some people like to have a wig on hand just in case, but I would recommend waiting to spend money on a wig, because in most people the hair loss is not severe enough to be noticeable by others.

• **"Cyclophosphamide can also suppress the bone marrow,** which is the organ where blood cells are manufactured. Suppression of the bone marrow can result in anemia, or low red-cell count; leucopenia, or low white-cell count; and thrombocytopenia, or low platelet count. Red cells carry oxygen through the circulation to the whole body, and anemia, if severe, can deprive body organs of enough oxygen for normal function. The most common symptoms of anemia are tiredness, lack of energy, and easy fatigability. White cells are important in the body's defense against infection, and leukopenia makes a person more susceptible to infections. Platelets are important in normal blood coagulation, and severe thrombocytopenia can lead to prolonged bleeding and poor clot formation."

Azathioprine

"Once the course of cyclophosphamide is completed, during which we will be reducing the dose of prednisone, we will start you on **oral azathioprine,**"the rheumatologist told Phyllis. "This drug also suppresses the immune system, but not as strongly as cyclophosphamide. Recent studies have shown that remissions induced by cyclophosphamide are maintained more effectively by taking a moderate dosage of azathioprine afterward. But azathioprine also has side effects:

• **"Azathioprine can suppress the bone marrow**, in much the same manner as cyclophosphamide, leading to anemia, leukopenia, and thrombocytopenia.

• **"Azathioprine can also have toxic effects on the liver**, and we will need to watch for signs of this by checking your blood for various sensitive tests of liver malfunction at regular intervals while you take this medication."

Phyllis commented,"I wonder if the treatment isn't worse than the disease!"

"I guess it can be, but I have focused on worst-case scenarios in discussing this with you. Usually, things go along well, and we don't run into any of these problems," observed the rheumatologist.

Phyllis asked,"How well does this treatment work?"

What benefit can I expect from treatment?

The rheumatologist, who was getting hoarse from talking by now, said, "In my experience, this is the best form of treatment that we have for lupus with severe kidney disease. We are trying to do two things—both keep you alive and preserve your kidneys. If we accomplish both of those goals, the treatment will have been successful. But in most cases, we also get pretty much a complete remission of the systemic disease, so the bothersome but not particularly dangerous symptoms you had at the beginning, including the arthritis, should be gone. We are also trying to do this without side effects, and we usually succeed.

"Nevertheless, sometimes we cannot totally control the disease, and it recurs. If this happens, we simply repeat the course of medications and try again. The risk of side effects is greater the second time around, but we still usually get by with it. But if this happens repeatedly, you could lose kidney function over time, possibly eventually resulting in the need for dialysis and kidney transplantation. That is certainly not the ideal outcome, but even patients who come to transplantation usually do very well, especially if the transplanted kidney comes from a living, related donor."

"Is kidney disease the worst thing this disease can do to me, or do you have other tricks up your sleeve?" asked Phyllis.

What else could SLE do to me?

"Well, severe kidney disease is one of several serious forms that lupus can take," began the rheumatologist. "Although SLE can cause problems in almost any system of the body, there are two other major problems that could arise, and we will be on the alert for them. Statistically, if they don't occur in the first couple of years, they become somewhat less likely ever to happen in a given person.

"If SLE affects the central nervous system, it can cause very severe problems, the most dramatic of which are strokes, convulsive seizures, and psychoses.

- "**Strokes** look just like the typical strokes that people can get with arteriosclerosis —hardening of the arteries—in which some neurological functions suddenly stop. One side of the body can become paralyzed, sometimes with loss of speech and some mental functions. This can lead to permanent disability, or if vital centers of the brain, especially the brain stem, are affected, a person could die. The big difference between these strokes and the more common variety is that lupus-induced strokes tend to occur in younger people.

- "**Seizures** can be total body convulsions (grand mal) or more limited (petit mal), in which the affected person may or may not recognize that something has happened. Either way, patients need to be treated with anticonvulsant medications.

- "**Psychosis** can take the form of any mental disorder, or it can look more like an organic brain syndrome, in which the person loses short-term memory and becomes disoriented.

"These neurological conditions vary in the degree to which they respond to standard SLE treatment, and in some cases there is disagreement about what the best treatment should be. Generally, they are treated with prednisone along with more specific therapy for the conditions they look like—that is, anticonvulsants for seizures or antipsychotic drugs for psychosis.

"**The other major condition occurs when antibodies form against components of the coagulation system.** Although these antibodies are commonly referred to as lupus anticoagulants, they do not typically cause bleeding. Paradoxically, **they cause trouble by activating the coagulation system so that clotting occurs spontaneously in the blood vessels, leading to blockage of the blood supply to the organs supplied by those blood vessels.** This may be what happens in at least some forms of SLE-induced strokes, but it can occur in almost any organ.

"This phenomenon appears to be responsible for spontaneous miscarriages in pregnant women with lupus. It is associated with fatal hemorrhagic pneumonia in lupus. It can cause deep vein thrombophlebitis, that is, blood clots in the leg veins, which can break off clots that go to the lungs, called pulmonary embolus, and other organs. It can result in disseminated intravascular coagulation—called DIC for short—with widespread gangrene caused by blockage of blood circulation in many vessels, an often-fatal condition. The modern name of this condition is **antiphospholipid syndrome**. The treatment for it is to recognize it before it causes problems by testing for antibodies against phospholipids—the typical one tested for is anticardiolipin—and treating aggressively with anticoagulants, usually warfarin. These antibodies often cause a false positive test for syphilis, which also uses the cardiolipin antigen.

"We have tested you for anticardiolipin antibodies, and none are detectable in your circulation, so I don't think you have to worry about this right now. But we need to stay vigilant," the doctor stressed.

"I asked you about pregnancy before, but I forgot to ask whether SLE is hereditary. Is it?" inquired Phyllis.

Is SLE hereditary?

"There appears to be a hereditary component in lupus. It tends to run in families. There is a 10 percent likelihood that a family member of a patient with lupus will also have it. There is a 69 percent likelihood that an identical twin of a lupus patient will also have it. Some hereditary antigens on white cells (HLA antigens A1, B8, DR2, DR3, and DQ1) are more common in SLE than in the population at large. But it is unlikely that genetics tells the whole story. It seems that some people inherit the susceptibility to SLE, but in reality, anyone can get it," answered the doctor.

Subsequent course

Phyllis tolerated the course of strong medicines the doctor prescribed for her. She gained about thirty pounds during the early going because of prednisone, but by two years later she was on a minimal dose of prednisone and azathioprine, and was back to her original weight. She felt well. She and Harold had gotten married, but they had decided to wait to start a family until Phyllis was off medications. That took another three years, during which she had no attacks of SLE, and her kidney function was normal.

Six years after the original attack, Phyllis and Harold decided that they had waited long enough. After consultation with Phyllis's doctor, who gave his blessing, they took the necessary steps and Phyllis became pregnant. A high-risk obstetrician recommended by her rheumatologist monitored her pregnancy, and after nine uneventful months, she gave birth to a beautiful seven-pound daughter that she and Harold named Hyacinth. Both the baby and the mother did fine. Phyllis continued to see her doctor at six-month intervals, and she and her family are doing well to this day.

Not everyone is so fortunate, as the high-risk obstetrician told Phyllis and Harold. By delaying pregnancy for so long after all signs of active lupus had abated, they had minimized but not eliminated the risk of a lupus flare. Even after many years of apparent quiescence, lupus can reactivate and be very difficult to control. But Phyllis, Harold, and Hyacinth (who is now in college) got through it unscathed, and that is what counts.

Disease at a glance: Systemic lupus erythematosus

Who gets it?

- Women seventeen to thirty-five years old, predominantly
- More frequent and more severe in African Americans
- Moderate heredity component
- At least 239,000 Americans affected

Joint involvement

- Small joints of hands and wrists most frequent
- Nondestructive arthritis
- Frequent avascular/aseptic necrosis (see glossary) of hips, knees, shoulders, especially with high-dose corticosteroid treatment
- Usually joints are not the main problem (see below)

Other features and complications

- Glomerulonephritis/kidney failure
- Convulsions or psychosis
- Pleurisy/pericarditis (serositis)
- Antiphospholipid syndrome
    - o Stroke
    - o Multiple miscarriages
    - o Hemorrhagic pneumonitis
- Skin rash (malar, or over-the-cheeks, distribution—called butterfly rash)
- Photosensitivity
- Hair loss
- Mouth ulcers

Laboratory features

- Anemia, low white-cell count, low platelet count
- Antinuclear antibody (ANA)
- Antibodies against DNA, other nuclear antigens
- False positive syphilis test (due to antiphospholipid antibodies)
- Protein and red-cell casts in the urine
- Low complement levels
- Elevated acute phase reactants

Treatment

- General
    - o Adequate rest
    - o Appropriate exercise
    - o Education
- Medications for arthritis and skin features
    - o Aspirin or other NSAID
    - o Antimalarial drug

- Medications for kidney and/or central nervous system features
  - o Systemic corticosteroids
  - o Systemic immunosuppressive drugs
- Other treatments as indicated for less common features

Chapter 9
Infectious Arthritis
Onset: What's a joint like this doing in a nice girl like you?

Frieda had just turned sixty-four, and she was looking forward to retiring the following year. After more than forty years of working as a maid and cleaning lady in the county hospital, she was about worn out. But she had a lot to be thankful for.

She had come to America from her childhood home in western Poland as a teenage orphan, speaking only German and Polish and with little education, minimal cash, and no prospects. She considered herself fortunate to have landed in a friendly, blue-collar, European immigrant community in a midwestern steel-manufacturing city. Through the church, she made some friends who spoke Polish and German, learned some English, and found work in the hospital.

She eventually met Jakob, a nice young steelworker only a couple of years older than she was. He and his parents had immigrated from a village a few miles east of Frieda's hometown. He courted her, and they married after a few months. One of the proudest days in both of their lives was the one when they became American citizens. Over the next five years, they had four children: two girls (Hannah and Hedwig) and two boys (Heinrich and Hermann).

Then, tragically, just after their tenth anniversary, when everything seemed to be going well, Jakob was killed in a freak accident at the plant. Although Jakob had only a small insurance policy, the company had a fairly liberal attitude about their obligations to families of employees injured or killed on the job, and they agreed to provide a stipend to Frieda, at least until her children were through school. This, together with her small salary from the hospital, enabled her to support the family. Frieda was very frugal, and she saved at least half of her salary. Mr. Drobkin at the bank advised her to put some of her money into securities, and he managed her account for her. The children got part-time jobs as soon as they were able and contributed to the household as well.

Eventually, all the children grew up, finished their educations, got jobs, got married, and moved to other cities, where there was greater opportunity for white-collar employment. None settled near Frieda, and to be honest, they were a little embarrassed by her accent and old-world ways. Heinrich became Henry, and Hedwig became Hedy. They joined country clubs, raised their own families, had their own problems, and seldom saw, talked to, or thought about their mother or one another.

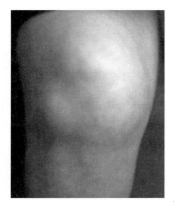

Figure 1: Swelling of a single knee (monoarthritis) is typical of infectious arthritis, although it may also be seen in several other conditions. In tuberculous arthritis, the inflammation is generally not as intense as in arthritis caused by pus-forming bacteria, like staph and strep.

Frieda continued working without complaint and putting her money away, and she was finally approaching retirement. One day, shortly after her sixty-fourth birthday, she noticed that her right knee was a little stiff and sore, and it looked mildly swollen. *Figure 1*. She figured she had twisted it while carrying her scrub bucket up three flights of stairs, as she did every day. But the swelling didn't go down, and it seemed to be getting a little worse as the weeks wore on. Frieda knew she was dependent on a reasonable degree of physical well-being in order to maintain her livelihood. Anything that looked as if it might limit her capacity to work was a significant threat, so she decided not to put off consulting a physician about the knee any longer. She knew some of the doctors in the rheumatology department at the hospital where she worked. She liked them all, but she knew that one, a woman, was fluent in German, and she sought her out.

Initial evaluation: What did the doctor say?

The doctor greeted Frieda warmly, and after a short conversation about her family, she asked her the reason for her visit. Frieda described the problem with her right knee. The doctor asked her many questions, emphasizing information about her general health and medical history, as well as any history of operations or injuries. Frieda had not had chills, fever, weight loss, or any other symptoms suggesting chronic illness. She had experienced some sweating at night and hot flashes since she stopped menstruating some fifteen years earlier. The doctor inquired in detail about Frieda's family medical history, but details were sketchy on this issue. Frieda couldn't remember much about her parents' health, and she had no brothers or sisters. She reported that her four children were all healthy and that her pregnancies had been uneventful.

Following this, the doctor examined Frieda carefully, paying particular attention to her skin; listening carefully to her lungs through the stethoscope; feeling for enlarged lymph nodes, liver, and spleen; checking all her joints; and manipulating the right knee. The examination was pretty much normal except for the obvious swelling in the right knee, which was also mildly tender and warmer to touch than the left knee. Throughout the examination, the doctor kept up a running commentary on what she was finding, and Frieda found that quite reassuring.

The doctor then proceeded to discuss her assessment of the situation and the next steps she recommended. Speaking in German, she said, "Frieda, you have a condition in the right knee that we rheumatologists refer to as monoarticular arthritis. That means that your arthritis affects only one joint. Most forms of arthritis affect several or many joints. While there are several conditions that can lead to monoarticular arthritis, the most likely causes are an infection in the joint or crystal-induced arthritis, like gout or pseudogout. Unfortunately, we do not have many useful leads from your medical history. The most straightforward approach to making the correct diagnosis is to remove some fluid from your knee through a needle, then examine it under the microscope and test it in the laboratory. We need to do this before starting any treatment."

Frieda was a little fearful about having a needle inserted into her knee, but she trusted the doctor and, after thinking about it for a couple of minutes, asked her to go ahead. The doctor left the room, returning a few minutes later with a nurse, whose name was Tyrone, carrying an instrument tray. Tyrone asked Frieda to lie down on the examining table and placed a rolled-up towel under her right knee, flexing it slightly.

The rheumatologist washed her hands and assumed her position on the left side of the examining table. Tyrone gave her a pair of rubber gloves, which she quickly put on. He then held out a packet with three iodine-soaked applicators, which the doctor took one at a time. She painted her gloved left index finger with the first one, and then painted Frieda's right knee three times with the brown solution, using all the applicators. Tyrone then held out another packet with a single applicator protruding. This one was soaked with alcohol, and the doctor painted her index finger and the knee with this solution. She probed the knee with the antiseptic-treated finger to find the best area to introduce the needle. Next, Tyrone produced a small syringe with a clear solution inside, and the doctor took it and injected it just beneath the skin at the upper, inner edge of the kneecap, raising a sizable welt.

"Ach, that burns!" exclaimed Frieda.

"It's just a little local anesthetic to make the area numb," explained the doctor in German. "It's normal to feel a little burning sensation during injection of this medicine."

Next, Tyrone produced a much bigger syringe with a long, pink-hubbed needle. Frieda looked on with horror and gripped the edges of the table as hard as she could. The doctor took the syringe and carefully introduced the needle a short distance through the skin. Frieda felt nothing, and she began to relax a little.

"Are we done?" Frieda inquired hopefully.

"Almost," said the doctor reassuringly. She then gave the needle a quick push into the knee joint. Frieda felt an instant sharp pain as the needle penetrated into the joint space, but there was no further pain. Frieda could see the syringe filling with a cloudy yellow liquid that looked like it was tinged with blood. The doctor removed several syringes full of this synovial (joint) fluid, placing small amounts into several sterile containers that would be used for culture and analysis of the fluid. Finally, the doctor removed the needle from the knee, and Tyrone immediately began to swab the skin over the knee and, after putting pressure on the needle site for a couple of minutes, placed a small bandage over the penetration site.

"All done," said the doctor. "That wasn't so bad, was it?"

"Not as bad as I expected, but bad enough," responded Frieda. Actually, the knee felt a little better after much of the excess fluid had been removed.

"Okay, Frieda, I think that's the best we can expect under the circumstances. While you are getting dressed, I'm going to take a look at the joint fluid under the microscope to look for the presence of crystals that would enable us to make a diagnosis of gout or pseudogout. Then we'll send you off for some blood tests and X-rays. Since your knee is not acutely painful, if I don't see any crystals, I think we can safely wait until we see the results of the testing before starting any treatment. Do you know if you have ever had a skin test for tuberculosis?"

"My skin test is positive because I had a BCG vaccination to prevent tuberculosis as a child in Poland," recalled Frieda.

The doctor knew that, beginning in the 1920s, vaccination with a TB-like bacterium called BCG (Bacillus Calmette-Guérin) was widely used in many countries to build immunity against tuberculosis. It is variably effective in preventing tuberculosis (from 0 to 76 percent in several studies), but it almost always causes the tuberculosis skin test to convert to positive, thus rendering it ineffective as a diagnostic test for tuberculosis. In the United States, the Centers for Disease Control and Prevention (CDC) do not recommend its routine use because of its variable effectiveness and the relatively low risk of contracting tuberculosis in this country. However, as this book is going to press, the CDC is revising the 1988 recommendations, which are currently in effect. For Frieda, however, the decision had already been made.

"Okay, we'll skip the skin test," said the doctor.

The microscopic examination of the joint fluid did not reveal any crystals, but many inflammatory cells were present. This was not surprising, since the knee had the characteristics that suggested a chronic inflammatory process—swelling and warmth.

Frieda went off to the lab for blood testing and to the X-ray department for knee and chest X-rays, and then she went back to work. She was very conscientious about working, and she would have to be a lot sicker than this to stay away from her job at the hospital.

The doctor's report

A week later, Frieda reported to the doctor's office to find out what the tests and X-rays showed and to hear the recommendations for treatment. Again, the doctor greeted her warmly, and after brief small talk, she got down to business.

"Frieda," she said in German, "you have tuberculous arthritis of the knee. The tuberculosis bacterium grew out of your joint fluid in the laboratory cultures, and it was also visible in the joint fluid under the microscope with special staining—an acid-fast stain—so there is no doubt about the diagnosis.

"Although we normally think of tuberculosis as a disease of the lungs," the doctor continued, "the germ that causes tuberculosis—*Mycobacterium tuberculosis*—can sometimes infect other tissues. The lungs are the most commonly affected organs because the usual way this germ gets into the body is by being inhaled. But in your case, the 'bug' settled in the right knee, and that appears to be the only site where it is now growing."

The doctor went on. "Because of the public health implications of tuberculosis, I will need to report your case to the health department, and they and I will share the responsibility for your treatment."

Frieda was shocked. "How can I have TB? This is America, and I haven't been around anyone with TB since I left the old country. Anyway, I was vaccinated against it when I was a child."

Frieda's Questions

How did I get this?

"In the first place," said the doctor, "you and I work in the county hospital, which serves the inner city. In this hospital, we take care of many people with deficient immune systems from AIDS and other conditions. Such individuals have an increased likelihood of becoming infected with tuberculosis, and they can pass it on to others, mainly by coughing. You go into many patients' rooms each day, and some of them may have tuberculosis that they don't even know about.

"Secondly, although tuberculosis is not as common in the United States as in many other countries, its frequency is on the rise here. That is a matter of concern to public health officials, especially since many of these cases, unlike in the past, are resistant to the usual forms of treatment.

"Finally, as you mentioned to me last week, you had BCG vaccination against TB as a child. Unfortunately, BCG vaccination is nowhere nearly as effective against TB as, say, smallpox vaccination is against smallpox or polio vaccination is against polio. And even when it is effective, the effectiveness tends to decline with the passage of time. You received BCG at least a half-century ago, and it clearly didn't prevent the infection that you now have. The main thing that BCG did for you is prevent you from participating in the hospital's TB surveillance program, which relies on annual skin tests for all employees. It might also have modified the way your body handled the TB germs, resulting in this unusual form of TB."

Frieda became thoughtful. "Just how contagious is this infection? Can people catch it from me? Am I going to lose my job?"

Am I contagious?

"Don't worry; you are not going to lose your job because of this," the doctor reassured Frieda. "You will need to stay off work until the knee joint responds to treatment. We don't want you to cause any unnecessary damage to the knee by overusing it while the arthritis is active.

"Although you have live, infectious TB germs in your body, considering their location in the right knee and the lack of evidence that they are anywhere else right now, and also considering that you are not coughing, it is not likely that you are spreading this disease around at present. Coughing is the main mode by which this disease spreads, and you probably got it by being around someone with TB who was coughing. Nevertheless, we have to start you on effective treatment, not only because of the damage the disease can cause to your knee, but also because you could become contagious in the future if the bacteria reenter your bloodstream and make their way back to the lungs. We certainly don't want that to happen."

Frieda then asked, "How did the TB get to my knee if it came into my body through my lungs?"

How did the infection get to my knee?

The doctor answered, "The main route from the lungs to the joints or any other organ is the bloodstream, and that's probably how it happened in your case. The most commonly affected joints are those of the spine—the joints between the bones of the spine are called intervertebral joints—the hips, and the knees. When TB goes to the intervertebral joints in the spine, it's called Pott's disease after Percivall Pott, an English barber-surgeon who described tuberculosis of the spine in the eighteenth century. An interesting sidelight is that one of Pott's pupils was John Hunter, a student of smallpox, whose observation that milkmaids seldom contracted smallpox led to Edward Jenner's pioneering use of the cowpox virus, or vaccinia, to vaccinate against smallpox.

"Another interesting question is when did the primary infection occur? Some people get lung TB, which becomes inactive or latent and sits there for many years without causing any problems. We can sometimes see this latent TB on a chest X-ray, where it appears as a calcified lesion called a Ghon focus, after Austrian pathologist Anton Ghon, who described it in 1912. Usually, this type of lesion doesn't progress, but occasionally, for unknown reasons, it activates and causes disease, either in the lungs or elsewhere. However, your chest X-ray showed no evidence of a Ghon focus or any other abnormality suggesting tuberculosis, so I suspect that the initial infection occurred here fairly recently."

"Why don't I have a fever?" asked Frieda. "I thought that when a person has an infection with bacteria there should be fever."

Why don't I have a fever?

"Actually, you may have had fever at times, and we may simply not have checked you at a time when your temperature was elevated," answered the doctor. "Sometimes, people infected with the tubercle bacillus have fever that isn't apparent to them. Not all fevers are accompanied by chills and shaking. The most common symptom of fever in people with tuberculosis is night sweats, and these tend to occur at the time the fever is breaking, that is, when the temperature is returning to normal. But some fevers are completely without symptoms, and the only way you can detect them is by taking the temperature with a thermometer. However, some people with localized tuberculosis do not have fever at all, and you may be one of them.

"Most other bacteria cause a more acute infection than the tubercle bacillus does. A joint infected with staphylococcus (staph for short) or streptococcus (strep for short), or some other pyogenic (pus-producing) infectious agent tends to be tightly swollen, extremely tender, and very warm to the touch. Such bacteria are all around us in our daily lives, but fortunately, most people avoid infection with them. People infected with these agents tend to have high fevers that remain elevated until they are treated with antibiotics. They also often have bacteria circulating in the blood, and cultures of blood can lead to growth of the bacteria in the laboratory. People with such infections may be acutely ill and show classical signs of sepsis, such as fever and rigors, up to and including shock if the blood pressure drops to subnormal levels. These infections tend to be rapidly destructive, and they must be treated as medical emergencies.

"Infectious funguses can also occasionally get into the joints and cause a form of arthritis that resembles tuberculous arthritis," the doctor explained. "They tend to get into the body either by inhalation or through breaks in the skin. They can make their way to the joints through the bloodstream. They're inflammatory, but the inflammation is usually of a lower grade than that caused by the pus-producing bacteria—it's subacute like tuberculosis, rather than acute like staph. Many of these agents are rather prevalent in the environment as well. Some, like *Histoplasma capsulatum*, the fungus that causes histoplasmosis, and *Coccidioides immitis*, the fungus that causes coccidioidomycosis, have characteristic geographic distributions. In the United States, histoplasmosis is commonest in the Tennessee, Ohio, and Mississippi valleys, and coccidioidomycosis is most frequent in the San Joaquin Valley. When they infect the joints, these funguses are identified by examination of joint fluid."

Frieda's head was spinning. She was hearing more about arthritis than she had ever wanted to know. But since she had the doctor to herself, at least for the moment, she was determined to find out everything she could about her condition. She asked, "Can this tuberculosis spread to my other joints?"

Can infectious arthritis affect multiple joints?

"That's a very perceptive question, Frieda, and the answer is that, fortunately, your TB is not very likely to spread to other joints," said the doctor. "Most joint infections involve only one joint. A few infectious agents, the most familiar being gonorrhea, can get into multiple joints, but that rarely happens in tuberculosis.

"There are some bacteria and viruses, nevertheless, that can cause arthritis that is not due to direct infection of the joints, but rather to a generalized reaction of the body against the infection, and this situation often leads to symptoms of arthritis in many joints. If you test the joint fluid from affected joints in such patients, the responsible infectious agent cannot be found there.

• "**Rheumatic fever arthritis** is the most familiar example of this type of arthritis. In this condition, the responsible germ is a bacterium called streptococcus. Rheumatic fever is caused by the body's immune reaction against this streptococcus, which usually infects the throat. Strep throat is not to be taken lightly because of the heart valve abnormalities that can result from this inappropriate autoimmune response. The immune system mistakes the body's own tissues for the streptococcus and attacks them as a part of its reaction against the strepto-coccus. This occurs because certain chemicals on the surface of the streptococcus mimic chemicals in the human body. This phenomenon is called molecular mimicry, and it is one of the mechanisms underlying autoimmunity. The arthritis of rheumatic fever is generally mild and fleeting, and does little or no harm to the joints.

• "**Tuberculosis** *may* **also cause an immunologically generated arthritis called Poncet's arthritis.** Antonin Poncet, a French surgeon, described it in 1897. It rarely occurs in people with tuberculosis, affects multiple joints, and may look like rheumatoid arthritis. This arthritis tends not to be destructive. The test for rheumatoid factor may be positive in such patients. No tubercle bacilli are found in the joint fluid, and the joint fluid is sterile, just as in rheumatic fever. Perhaps because this condition is very rare and would be found primarily in places where tuberculosis is common, American and British physicians are unsure that it exists. Since rheumatoid arthritis is also relatively common, the co-occurrence of these two diseases—tuberculosis and rheumatoid arthritis—in the same individual would be expected to occur occasionally, and I suppose this could be an explanation for what we call Poncet's arthritis."

Frieda exclaimed, "*Gott im Himmel*, enough already! Can you cure this?"

What's the treatment, and how likely is it to succeed?

The doctor responded in German, "**We should be able to cure the tuberculosis in the knee using a combination of joint drainage and antibiotics specific for tuberculosis.** The drug treatments we have now are very effective and remarkably safe as well. But if the infection has caused any damage to the joint, the antituberculous treatment will not cure that. **If there is any residual joint damage, we will have to treat it the way we treat osteoarthritis.**

"We'll drain the excess fluid from the knee weekly for the first few weeks or as long as fluid continues to accumulate and the knee remains swollen. We'll do it just the way we did to get the sample for joint fluid analysis. This allows the antibiotics to get into the knee better and makes them more effective.

"As in other infectious diseases, the medical treatment for tuberculosis has changed over time, and it's almost certain to continue to change as new antibiotics are developed and as tubercle bacilli continue to evolve new drug-resistant strains. In 2003, the federal government's Centers for Disease Control and Prevention—the CDC—along with the American Thoracic Society and the Infectious Diseases Society of America, promulgated the current evidence-based guidelines for treatment, and these are what we use today to treat tuberculosis of the lungs, or pulmonary TB, and other organs, including the joints, that is, extrapulmonary TB."

The doctor outlined the **four-drug therapy.** "**We will start with four antituberculous drugs: isoniazid, or INH; rifampin, or RIF; pyrazinamide, or PZA; and ethambutol, or EMB.** Fortunately, these drugs come in combination preparations, so it will only be necessary for you to keep track of a few pills. For example, Rifamate is a combination of INH and RIF, and Rifater is a combination of INH, RIF, and PZA. All four drugs are necessary at first, because we don't yet know whether your particular TB germ is resistant to INH, as is frequently the case. We refer to this as four-drug therapy for obvious reasons. We will find out how long we have to continue this four-drug therapy from testing the bacterium that grew out of your joint fluid against INH and the other drugs. This is called sensitivity testing. Once we have the sensitivity test results from your knee-joint fluid cultures, we can decide which of the drugs you actually need going forward. If your TB germ is sensitive to INH and RIF, we will be able to stop the EMB," concluded the doctor.

"How long do I have to take these drugs?" asked Frieda.

What is the duration of treatment?

"There are two parts, or phases, to the treatment," answered the doctor, " the initiation phase, during which treatment is more intensive, lasting for eight weeks; and the continuation phase, during which treatment is reduced, lasting for twenty-six weeks. The total treatment takes about eight months, assuming that everything goes according to plan. As I mentioned, we will begin the initiation phase with four-drug therapy, but we may be able to go to three-drug therapy when we get the sensitivity results."

"Do I have to be in the hospital?" asked Frieda.

"No, but I will need to see you fairly frequently in the office, both to track your response to treatment and to make sure that you are not having side effects from the drugs," replied the doctor.

"Can I work?" asked Frieda.

"Once your knee has stopped swelling, assuming that you are still not coughing, you can return to work," answered the doctor.

"I never heard of any of these drugs. Do they have side effects?" asked Frieda dubiously.

What are the side effects of treatment?

"**These drugs, like all drugs, have side effects**," the doctor told Frieda. "Although many side effects are possible, they are not particularly frequent with any of these drugs.

- INH can cause skin rash, stomach upset, side effects in the liver and the nervous system, and deficiency of the vitamin pyridoxine.

- RIF can cause stomach upset, side effects in the liver and the kidneys, low platelet count, visual disturbances, menstrual irregularities, and swelling of the face and extremities.

- EMB can cause visual disturbances, skin rashes, itching, joint pain, gout, and side effects in the liver and kidneys.

- PZA can cause stomach upset, joint pain, hives and itching, gout, and side effects in the liver.

"Like most drugs, all four of these can cause allergic reactions in people who happen to be hypersensitive to them. We have to watch for these reactions, but I would emphasize that these drugs are pretty safe, as long as we monitor them closely. Fortunately, if it turns out that we can't use one or more of them, there are quite a few alternatives to pick from."

"I am almost afraid to ask this, but what if I had a different kind of infection in a joint? How different would the treatment be?" asked Frieda.

What is the treatment for other forms of infectious arthritis?

"The principles of treating infectious arthritis are the same regardless of the type of infection," replied the doctor, warming to the topic. "The goals of treatment are always to cure the infection and minimize or prevent damage to the infected joint. That means that the sooner we get an accurate diagnosis and start the treatment, the better off we are.

"The tools of treatment are (a) protection of the infected joint by draining the inflammatory fluid as often as necessary and (b) getting rid of the infection by administration of the proper antibiotics in full dosage, by the most efficient route— by mouth, intravenously, or injection into muscle—and for the appropriate length of time. In many infections, although not in tuberculosis, the antibiotics must be given intravenously, or IV. This generally starts in the hospital, although we use home antibiotic infusions after the acute phase of the infection is controlled and we are certain that the infection is responding to treatment."

Treatment begins

"So, let's get started," suggested the doctor. "We will have you take the medications here daily for the next eight weeks. I will give you your first dose now, and Tyrone will have your medicines ready for you to take by mouth each day when you come in. **We will ask you to take these medications here so that we can verify, for the record, that you actually take them. This is called directly observed therapy, or DOT, and it is the standard method of treating tuberculosis and other diseases considered public health risks."**

The doctor called in nurse Tyrone, and he assisted her in withdrawing fluid from Frieda's bad knee with a needle and syringe and gave Frieda the first doses of the four antituberculous drugs. She then asked Frieda to return the next day to see Tyrone to get her medications, and in one week to see her for recheck and further joint drainage if necessary.

First follow-up visit and subsequent course

Frieda stayed home, as instructed, except for her daily visit to Tyrone. She liked Tyrone, but she had a hard time communicating with him in her broken English. He liked her, too, and he offered to bring the medications to her home so that she wouldn't have to come in to the hospital every day while she was supposed to be staying off her bad knee.

At Frieda's first follow-up visit with the rheumatologist, the knee was still swollen and a little tender. The doctor, aided by Tyrone, drained the knee again, but the volume of fluid she was able to get from the knee was about half what she had obtained before the onset of treatment. She noted that the sensitivity tests had shown that the germ infecting Frieda's knee was fully sensitive to INH, and she discontinued the EMB, leaving Frieda on INH, RIF, and PZA, thereby reducing her from quadruple to triple therapy.

On his daily visits, Tyrone noticed that Frieda's house needed some minor repairs, and he began to stay longer on Saturdays to fix some of these problems. As he put it, "Hey, I did this kind of stuff all the time for my mom before she died. I enjoy it." Frieda was very appreciative and made cookies and pies for him every weekend.

Meanwhile, her knee was getting better. The swelling had gone down completely by the fifth week of treatment, and the rheumatologist no longer needed to drain fluid from the knee. The X-rays showed only minimal damage to the knee joint, and the doctor said that Frieda could return to work on a light schedule.

When she reached the eight-week point, which concluded the initial phase of her treatment, the doctor told her that she was ready to begin the continuation phase. The doctor collected a sputum sample to test for TB germs, reduced the number of drugs from three to two—INH and a longer-acting form of RIF called rifapentine, or RPT—and reduced the frequency of administration from once daily to once weekly. The sputum sample was negative, and the doctor told Frieda that the continuation phase of treatment would last for eighteen weeks, after which she would not need further treatment.

About six weeks into the continuation phase, Tyrone arrived with her weekly dose of medications, but he was not alone. With him was his girlfriend, Latoya, and he happily announced to Frieda that they were going to get married. After that, Latoya came along on each of Tyrone's DOT medication visits. She was a bright, outgoing, attractive young woman, also a nurse, and Frieda thought the two of them made a terrific couple. Tyrone and Latoya asked Frieda to come to their wedding and fill the role of mother of the groom in the absence of his deceased mother. He said his mother would have wanted it that way. Frieda almost cried as she accepted the honor; none of her own kids had cared whether she was even present at their weddings, let alone played a significant role in them.

A few weeks after completing her course of antituberculous therapy, Frieda took stock of her situation with respect to her pending retirement. Because she had lived so frugally, putting away most of her small salary over the years, she was in pretty good shape financially. She would be able to start collecting Social Security in a few more months and would be able to live reasonably comfortably without working at a regular job. Tyrone and Latoya were about to become parents, and Frieda looked forward to playing with her adoptive grandchild. She even started a college fund for the as-yet-unborn baby. And so, that is how Frieda not only got rid of her tuberculosis with minimal damage to her knee, but also acquired a new family in the process.

Tuberculosis lore

Tuberculosis has been recognized as a disease under a variety of names for more than five thousand years. Hippocrates (460–377 BC) wrote that it was the most widespread disease of the time. However, its recognition as an infectious disease was considerably more recent. In his book *De Contagione et Contagiosis Morbis*, published in 1546, Girolamo Fracastoro pointed out that healthy people could contract the disease by being around individuals known to have it, and that it could even be passed on through handling of bed linens used by affected individuals. But almost another three and a half centuries passed before the germ that causes tuberculosis was identified. In 1882, Robert Koch proved that *Mycobacterium tuberculosis* was the culprit.

Attempts to develop a vaccine to prevent the disease culminated in the work of Calmette and Guérin in France. Inspired by Jenner's work with cowpox as a preventive for smallpox, they worked with a bacterium related to the tubercle bacillus called *Mycobacterium bovis* that, like cowpox, primarily caused disease in cattle. They were able to produce a version of this bacterium (called BCG) that was generally not harmful to humans but conferred some degree of immunity against tuberculosis. As noted previously, BCG was first used in humans in 1921. Unfortunately, the preparation was not standardized, and different versions of it were extremely variable in effectiveness. BCG is still used in some parts of the world, but not in the United States, and Frieda had received it in Poland as a child.

Nevertheless, after Koch's discovery of *Mycobacterium tuberculosis*, another six decades passed before scientists developed effective medications to combat the disease—streptomycin in 1943, para-aminosalicylic acid (PAS) in 1946, isoniazid (INH) in 1951, pyrazinamide (PZA) in 1954, cycloserine in 1955, ethambutol (EMB) in 1962, and rifampin (RIF) in 1963. Along the way, many well-known individuals were lost to the disease, including Russian author Anton Chekhov, Polish composer and musician Frédéric Chopin, French physician René-Théophile-Hyacinthe Laennec (inventor of the stethoscope), Czech novelist Franz Kafka, English poet John Keats, Scottish author Robert Louis Stevenson, and many members of the Brontë family.

Among the ineffective treatments advocated before the mid-twentieth century were bloodletting, laying on of hands by the king, gold therapy (later used in a somewhat less hazardous form for rheumatoid arthritis), collapse of one (or both!) lung(s), and the safer but just as ineffective sanatorium stay. Diagnosis was greatly aided by development of the chest X-ray in the nineteenth century and, of course, by cultures of sputum and other body fluids after Koch's discovery of the tubercle bacillus.

Sanatoriums were popular in the early twentieth century in Europe and the United States. They served the dual purpose of secluding tuberculosis patients from the general population and of providing peaceful settings in which they could while away their time waiting for the inevitable end, sort of an early version of palliative care. These sanatoriums were luxurious spas, especially in Europe, and they tended to be located in mountainous areas, where the air was considered to be more healthful than that in densely populated centers. That may have been true, but it was too late for the unfortunate sanatorium patients. Nevertheless, a rich social life flourished in these settings even as the residents were dying—fascinatingly documented by the German novelist Thomas Mann in his novel *The Magic Mountain* and in several short stories, all with sad endings. In the United States, most of these facilities closed after drug treatment of tuberculosis became possible. In Europe, however, the sanatoriums have become spas where people of means go for tune-ups and relaxation and to seek relief from various rheumatic and other ailments—or just to take a healthful vacation.

Today, the worldwide prevalence of tuberculosis has once again increased to the point where it has become an important public health problem, abetted by the AIDS epidemic. People with AIDS are more easily infected than people without AIDS, and they have become an unwilling reservoir for tuberculosis that is resistant to the commonly used antituberculous drugs. Fortunately, at least for now, there are some alternative drugs that can be used, but the need for careful adherence to accepted treatment protocols has never been greater. That is why the World Health Organization (WHO) and the Centers for Disease Control and Prevention strongly recommend the directly observed therapy approach described in Frieda's case.

Disease at a glance: Infectious arthritis

Who gets it?

- Anybody

Joint involvement

- Usually a single joint (monoarticular arthritis)
- Usually (not always) very painful, swollen, red, warm

Other features and complications

- Fever may or may not be present
- Often rapidly destructive
- Frequently superimposed on another form of arthritis, e.g., rheumatoid arthritis

Laboratory features

- Positive culture of joint fluid
- Blood culture *may* be positive
- Acute phase reactants *may* be elevated
- Joint fluid often has very high white-cell count

Treatment

- Education
- Joint drainage, usually surgical
- Systemic antibiotics (ATB)
  - o Broad-spectrum ATB until organism identified
  - o Appropriate specific ATB after organism identified
  - o Adequate dose and duration of treatment
- Reconstructive surgery (if needed) after the infection is cured

Chapter 10

Enteropathic (Inflammatory Bowel Disease) Arthritis

Onset: Rumbling in the back passage

Edgar Twickenham was a fastidious young man. As an accountant, he was the ultimate model of well-organized efficiency. No one in the finance department had a neater desk or a tidier cubicle. His grooming was immaculate, his dress shirts were spotless and well starched, the white handkerchief in his jacket pocket was carefully folded, his trousers were sharply creased, and his shoes were shined perfectly. He never wore socks that didn't match. The only things missing in his wardrobe were sleeve garters and green eyeshades.

Edgar took good care of himself and prided himself that his health was good. His only problems were long-standing constipation and, for the past few months, some aching and stiffness in the wrists and elbows. Sometimes his knees bothered him, but he was able to get reasonable relief by taking two or three ibuprofen capsules a few times daily during such periods.

Edgar was scrupulously courteous and professional in all his interpersonal relationships, especially at his place of employment. He never used first names; it was always Mr. This and Miss That. His work was beyond reproach to a degree that made his supervisor, Felix—sorry, Mr. Flatt—a mere mortal like most of the rest of us, a little uncomfortable. As Mr. Flatt always said, "When Edgar—I mean, Mr. Twickenham—counts the beans, they stay counted."

So, you can imagine Edgar's embarrassment when, one day, without any particular warning, he began to have uncontrollable flatulence at irregular but increasingly frequent intervals. These were not just quiet, easily ignored passages of small amounts of rapidly dispersed gas, but great, thunderous, odoriferous expulsions that commanded the attention and overwhelmed the senses of all in the office. Miss Perkins, Edgar's young assistant, herself a bit tightly wound, wrinkled her nose, pursed her lips, breathed shallowly, and pretended not to notice. On the other hand, many of their co-workers soon found a need to run errands in other parts of the building. Felix wondered, whimsically, if Edgar had been counting his beans and eating them, too.

To compound his mortification, Edgar began to feel an increasing urgency in his situation. Contrary to the satisfaction that one might reasonably expect from the elimination of large, unwanted volumes of intestinal gas, his bowels were suddenly seized with cramping pains such as he had never before experienced. Abandoning dignity, he sprang from his desk chair and, gripping his abdomen and shouting, "Look out, look out!" he ran for the men's room. It was just down the hall, and he almost made it in time. But just as he was crashing into the lone empty stall, he lost control, and—well, you can imagine the rest. Within moments, the other stalls hastily emptied out, and, alone at last, with some relief, he began to clean up.

To Edgar's horror, as if things were not bad enough, he noticed that, mixed in with the unformed bowel movement that he had produced a few minutes before, there were large amounts of what appeared to be blood in the stool. Now, in addition to the drained sensation that followed his explosive attack of diarrhea, Edgar was frightened. What in the world was going on? Other than chronic constipation, he had always been healthy, never had an ulcer, not even hemorrhoids. Yet in and around the toilet was what seemed to him to be a large amount of dark red blood.

It was not in Edgar's nature to procrastinate, and as soon as he was moderately presentable, he took himself to the local hospital's emergency room. Felix drove him (in Edgar's previously spotless car, a minivan with leather seats) and stayed with him, and Miss Perkins followed along in her VW, to provide additional support. The emergency-room doctor inserted an intravenous line and quickly decided that Edgar needed to be admitted to the hospital for intravenous fluids and possibly blood transfusion, as well as evaluation and control of gastrointestinal bleeding.

When he was ready to be wheeled off to his room, Edgar turned to Felix and Miss Perkins, and with uncharacteristic emotion in his voice, he croaked, "Miss Perkins, Mr. Flatt, thank you from the bottom of my heart for your support. I don't know what I would have done or how I would have gotten through all this without you here. Miss Perkins, I don't even know your first name, but you and Mr. Flatt are the best friends a fellow could want. I will never forget what you have done for me today. I'm pretty sure that I couldn't have done for anyone what you did for me."

Miss Perkins replied, blushing slightly, "You're welcome, Mr. Twickenham, and you may feel free to call me Twyla."

To make a long story short, Edgar was in the hospital for three days, during which he had the most comprehensive set of examinations he had ever experienced. It seemed to Edgar that his every orifice was probed and explored, every blood test was performed, and every X-ray was taken. During a colonoscopy (direct video examination of the colon using a small camera introduced through a flexible tube, called a colonoscope), multiple biopsies (tissue specimens) were taken. **After all these tests, the doctor, a gastroenterologist, told Edgar that he had Crohn's disease, an inflammatory disease of the intestinal wall, and that he would need to be on medications for it.**

How did the doctor know the diagnosis?

The doctor explained to Edgar that his case was somewhat unusual in that Crohn's disease usually starts with abdominal pain, poor appetite, and weight loss, rather than bloody diarrhea. Nonetheless, the diagnosis was confirmed by microscopic examination of a tissue specimen (biopsy) obtained during the colonoscopy, and there was no doubt about the diagnosis. In addition, the doctor thought that the joint pains Edgar had been experiencing might be related to the Crohn's disease. He noted that **a form of arthritis, often called enteropathic arthritis or IBD (inflammatory bowel disease) arthritis, is the most common nongastrointestinal complication of Crohn's disease, occurring in about 25 percent of cases.** He indicated that it was likely that this arthritis would improve as the inflammatory process in the intestine responded to treatment.

"Doctor, I have never heard of Crohn's disease. What is it?" asked Edgar.

Edgar's Questions

What is Crohn's disease?

"Crohn's disease is one form of inflammatory bowel disease," replied the doctor. "There are basically two types of disease—other than infections—that result from chronic inflammation in the wall of the intestines. These are both referred to generically as inflammatory bowel disease, or IBD. Ulcerative colitis, which mainly affects the large intestine, or colon, is one of them, and Crohn's disease, which affects both the small and large intestines, is the other. In Crohn's disease, the inflammation has a particular appearance under the microscope that pathologists call granulomatous inflammation. This type of inflammation, which also occurs in tuberculosis, has more or less round aggregations of cells typically found in chronic inflammation— as distinguished from acute inflammation—and central areas of dead tissue, called central necrosis. Recognition of these granulomatous areas is how pathologists can distinguish Crohn's disease from ulcerative colitis, which is not characterized by granuloma formation.

"Crohn's disease is named after Dr. Burrill B. Crohn, a specialist in gastrointestinal diseases, who described it in 1932 in a paper co-authored with two of his colleagues, Dr. Leon Ginzburg and Dr. Gordon Oppenheimer. All three worked together at Mount Sinai Hospital in New York City. They found and described fourteen patients with this form of inflammatory bowel disease. They called it regional ileitis because it most frequently affected the third part of the small intestine, called the ileum. Dr.

Crohn initially didn't believe that this disease ever affected the large intestine, but later he became convinced that it could. In fact, it can occur anywhere in the gastrointestinal tract, including the esophagus.

"Crohn's disease usually begins in people between the ages of twenty-five and forty, and it occurs in both men and women. It sometimes even affects children. It is more common in those who live in the Northern Hemisphere, who have relatively higher socioeconomic status, and who smoke. Although it can cause bloody diarrhea, as it did in your case," the doctor told Edgar, "it frequently starts with abdominal pain, constipation, and weight loss. Fever is often present. There are some very nasty things that it can do, including the formation of a connection, or fistula, between the lower intestine and the urinary bladder, the vagina, or the skin around the anus, with drainage of bowel contents through this fistulous tract."

"What does this have to do with arthritis?" Edgar asked.

What is the connection between Crohn's disease and arthritis?

"**Crohn's disease is one of many diseases that can have arthritis as a symptom.** Although it is pretty clear in Crohn's disease that the gastrointestinal component is the primary disease, in many other diseases, it can be hard to tell whether arthritis or some other component of the disease is primary. Systemic lupus erythematosus, for example, may start off looking like rheumatoid arthritis or juvenile chronic arthritis. Sometimes the primary disease takes a while to declare itself and leaves everybody scratching their heads until the disease is fully expressed. This can take months in some cases. This rarely happens with Crohn's disease, however.

"As I mentioned to you previously, **arthritis is the most common complication of Crohn's disease outside of the gastrointestinal tract. Arthritis, in fact, occurs in about 25 percent of people with Crohn's disease. When it does, the arthritis is called enteropathic arthritis or IBD arthritis.**

"There are at least two types of enteropathic arthritis:

- "The more common form is what you have, affecting one or more large joints of the extremities—elbows, wrists, knees, ankles. Less commonly, it can also affect the small joints of the hands as rheumatoid arthritis does. **In some ways, this form of enteropathic arthritis resembles rheumatoid arthritis**, but unlike rheumatoid arthritis, the rheumatoid factor test tends to be negative. [See chapter 2, page 9.] This arthritis features swelling of the affected joint or joints, with stiffness, warmth, and tenderness. There is often a tendency for much of the soreness to be around, rather than within, the affected joints, and this is referred to as periarticular inflammation. It usually doesn't cause permanent damage to the joints. Moreover, it tends to be active when the intestinal component of the disease is active and quiet when the intestines are quiet. Good control of the intestinal inflammation of Crohn's disease tends to keep this arthritis in check.

• "**The other type of enteropathic arthritis closely resembles ankylosing spondylitis.** It mainly involves the joints of the spine and the sacroiliac joints. In this condition, the inflammatory activity in the joints does not necessarily parallel that in the intestine. It can cause joint damage similar to that which occurs in primary ankylosing spondylitis (as described in chapter 5, page 51). People who get this form of enteropathic arthritis often have the HLA-B27 antigen, just as do those who have primary ankylosing spondylitis. We have to treat this type of arthritis independently of the intestinal disease, and control of the latter doesn't necessarily help the former, or vice versa."

"What causes this disease?" inquired Edgar.

What is the cause of Crohn's disease?

The doctor replied, "Crohn's disease may be associated, at least in some people, with genetically determined abnormalities in the immune system that allow the intestinal wall to be attacked by bacteria that normally inhabit the intestine. Specifically, in 2001, scientists found frequent mutations of the NOD2 gene, one of the genes controlling an early-warning system that indicates the presence of bacterial proteins in the cells of the intestinal wall in people with Crohn's disease. This may allow intestinal bacteria, which ordinarily would not be harmful, to attack the intestinal wall and set off the inflammatory mechanisms that cause the disease. If this is true, it opens the door for consideration of some sort of gene therapy for Crohn's disease in the future. But whether NOD2 mutation is the primary problem or even a significant problem in the mechanism of Crohn's disease is certainly not clear at this time. And it really doesn't directly explain the arthritis, which in this scenario would probably be reactive, that is, caused by remote inflammation.

"But other causes have been suggested, including viruses—such as the measles virus, for instance—and bacteria not normally found in the intestine. One such bacterium that has come under suspicion is *Mycobacterium paratuberculosis*. Involvement of this type of bacterium, related to the tuberculosis organism, could explain the granulomatous appearance of the intestinal biopsy in Crohn's disease.

"**The bottom line is that we really don't yet know for sure what causes Crohn's disease, but we strongly suspect that an immunological mechanism, possibly** such as the one I just described, is at the heart of the matter. The suspicion that the mechanism is an autoimmune one—immune reaction against one's own tissues—remains strong and is the basis for most of the treatments for Crohn's disease.

"One thing that seems certain is that Crohn's disease is not caused by dietary deficiencies or psychological stresses."

Edgar posed his next question, "You said that arthritis is the most common complication of Crohn's disease that occurs outside of the gastrointestinal tract, but what are the other complications?"

What are the other complications of Crohn's disease?

"Inside the gastrointestinal tract, the two most common complications are intestinal obstruction and fistulous tract formation," began the doctor.

- "**Intestinal obstruction** is an acute emergency, requiring hospitalization and often a surgical approach. Symptoms are severe abdominal pain, vomiting, abdominal distension, and no passage of gas via the rectum.

- "A **fistulous tract** is a tunnel that originates in an inflamed portion of the intestine and works its way either to the skin, generally around the anal area, or to the inside of a hollow organ, like the urinary bladder or the vagina. This allows passage of bowel contents through the fistula. If this material gets into the urinary bladder, it is certain to cause an infection in that organ. **Such fistulous tracts usually have to be removed surgically. Crohn's disease, allowed to remain active, may lead to intestinal cancer.**

- "Besides arthritis, Crohn's disease may be complicated by skin eruptions, gallstones, liver disease, or eye inflammation. Fortunately, at this point, you don't have any of these problems. They are not really uncommon, but they are less frequent than enteropathic arthritis. The connection of each of these complicating conditions with the underlying gastrointestinal disease remains poorly understood. Genetic factors might play a role. But this is not a nice disease."

"Is there a cure for Crohn's disease?" asked Edgar hopefully.

Can Crohn's disease be cured?

"Unfortunately, the answer is no," replied the doctor apologetically. "But we can treat it much more successfully now than in the past. Like many incurable inflammatory diseases, Crohn's disease is usually characterized by periods of activity, called exacerbations or flares, separated by periods of relative quiescence, called remissions.

"Dietary treatment is not very effective, but we generally recommend that people with active Crohn's disease follow a low-residue, low-fiber diet. This may lessen the stress on the intestinal tract by reducing the bulk of material that it has to handle, and by this mechanism, it may help minimally. More importantly, it is necessary to make sure that the diet is well balanced and has the right mix of vitamins and minerals, and this is especially relevant in the face of significant diarrhea.

"Over the years, many medications have been used, and several are effective. All of our drug treatments are aimed at reducing the inflammation in the intestinal wall. Some work directly against inflammation by one mechanism or another; others work against presumed causes of inflammation, such as bacterial infection or autoimmunity. The surgeon also has a role in treating some patients.

"The current treatment guidelines take into account the location, severity, and level of activity of the disease as well as the range of complications that are present. Because your disease was very active when you entered the hospital, Edgar, we started you on the best medication we have for quickly reducing inflammation and settling down an acute flare—prednisone. You have already made great strides, and as we are gradually reducing the dose of prednisone, we will now be starting maintenance treatment. Because you do not have intestinal obstruction or fistulous tracts, we do not for the present need the services of a surgeon.

"Maintenance drug treatment for Crohn's disease will include the use of an aminosalicylate, and for this we will use mesalamine. These anti-inflammatory medications can be tolerated for longer periods of time than the corticosteroid prednisone. But they are not as strong, and if the disease flares up again as prednisone is discontinued, we might have to supplement them with other medications, such as the immunosuppressive drugs azathioprine or methotrexate or the antibiotics metronidazole or ciprofloxacin. Recently, the very strong anti-inflammatory drug infliximab has been found effective, both in aiding prednisone in the induction of an initial remission and in supplementing the aminosalicylates in maintaining a remission. So as you can see, Edgar, we have a lot of arrows in our quiver when it comes to attacking this disease."

"That's great. But when I hear the word 'drugs,' I automatically think 'side effects.' What are they and how bad are they?" asked Edgar.

What are the side effects of treatment for Crohn's disease?

"That is a great question," acknowledged the doctor. "All these drugs have multiple side effects, and they are potentially severe if we don't monitor for them, discover them early when they occur, and take steps to minimize their results.

"**Prednisone** probably has a larger variety of potentially serious side effects than any of the other drugs, and that is why we use it sparingly and stop it as soon as we can. It can cause increased susceptibility to infection; weight gain; loss of bone calcium, or osteoporosis; diabetes; high blood pressure; fluid retention; mental and emotional aberrations; cataracts; and acne. Generally, however, for the short-term use of it to shut down a flare-up of the disease, most of these would be very unlikely. The big problems with prednisone in Crohn's disease tend to occur if we can't get a person off the drug and onto a reasonable maintenance program.

"**Mesalamine—and other salicylates**—can cause diarrhea, headache, abdominal pain, flatulence, malaise, fatigue, and nausea. You will probably notice that some of these side effects sound a lot like what you experienced with your initial attack of Crohn's disease. Although none of these is particularly dangerous, the occurrence of any of them could indicate either that the drug is ineffective or that it is causing a side effect. Either way, we would need to stop the drug, so the exact mechanism becomes something of a moot point.

"**Azathioprine** is an immunosuppressive drug that was used extensively in the early days of organ transplantation to prevent immune rejection. We now have much stronger and better—though more toxic—drugs for that purpose, but azathioprine is still used to treat certain autoimmune conditions these days, and its use in Crohn's disease is based on the theory, by no means proven, that autoimmunity plays a role in this condition. The side effects of azathioprine include low white blood-cell count resulting in reduced resistance to infection, anemia, low platelet count with increased risk of bleeding, and damage to the liver.

"Azathioprine also has significant drug interactions with allopurinol, a drug used to treat gout; warfarin, an anticoagulant drug used to prevent blood clotting; and blood -pressure drugs that work by inhibiting the angiotensin-converting enzyme, or ACE inhibitors.

"**Methotrexate**, also used to treat rheumatoid arthritis and certain other rheumatic diseases, can cause anemia, low white blood-cell count with increased susceptibility to infection, low platelet count with increased risk of bleeding, damage to the liver, pneumonia, nausea, and drowsiness. (See chapter 2, page 16-17, for more information about methotrexate.)

"**Metronidazole** is an antibiotic. It can cause neurological symptoms, including neurological pain—peripheral neuropathy—or seizures. It also can interact adversely with warfarin, phenobarbital, and phenytoin, an antiseizure medication.

"**Ciprofloxacin** is also an antibiotic. It can cause seizures, bloody diarrhea, tendon ruptures, and allergic rashes. It can interact adversely with warfarin and certain other drugs.

"**Infliximab** is a new 'biological' drug that suppresses inflammation by inhibiting the important mediator known as tumor necrosis factor-alpha, or TNF-alpha (see chapter 2, page 19). It is generally given intravenously, but there is interest in its effects on Crohn's disease when administered by mouth. Infliximab can reduce resistance to infection and even lower the white blood-cell count. There is also some evidence that infliximab can increase the likelihood of developing a lymphoma, a type of malignancy affecting the lymph nodes. Some people have allergic reactions to infliximab, and occasionally people have had lupuslike reactions, with rash, arthritis, and positive tests for antinuclear antibodies. People with demyelinating diseases—which attack the myelin coating, which insulates and protects nerve fibers—of the central nervous system, like multiple sclerosis, can be made worse by infliximab, and the drug should be avoided or used with great caution in this setting."

"You mentioned surgery. What are we talking about there?" asked Edgar.

What is the role of surgery?

"There are some situations where surgery is necessary on an emergency basis. If the intestine perforates, releasing intestinal contents into the abdominal cavity, that is a disaster that quickly leads to peritonitis, sepsis, and death unless emergency surgery is performed. Intestinal obstruction that does not resolve with placement of a tube into the intestine may also require surgery. Finally, persistent activity of the disease in spite of drug treatment may require a surgical approach.

"If an operation is necessary, the surgeon generally removes the section of the intestine that is inflamed. Depending on how much intestine has to be removed, this can have long-term consequences for nutrition. The small intestine is normally twelve to twenty feet in length. If a large portion of the intestine has to be removed, leaving less than five feet of small intestine if the colon has to be removed or less than two feet of small intestine if the colon is preserved, a person may need total parenteral nutrition, that is, all nutrition given intravenously. This is called short-bowel syndrome. Sometimes the surgical procedure requires the temporary or permanent rerouting of the end of the intestine to the surface of the abdomen—colostomy or ileostomy, depending on the part of the intestine at the orifice—and the use of a bag to collect the fecal material."

Edgar responded, "Well, that doesn't sound ideal. How well do the drugs work?"

What is the likely outcome of treatment?

The doctor thought for a few moments, looked a little uncomfortable, and then said, "For the acute episode, the drugs—especially prednisone—tend to work pretty well. Most people get a very nice response initially. But Crohn's disease is a chronic condition, and it tends to relapse after periods of remission, even in the face of fairly aggressive treatment. Unfortunately, none of the drugs we have now can keep the disease in remission permanently, and we usually need to go back to prednisone, either alone or in combination with one or more other drugs, from time to time to restore order. If the disease becomes intractable and doesn't respond to drug therapy, then we need to call the surgeon.

"With respect to your enteropathic arthritis, generally no specific antiarthritic treatment is necessary, because the arthritis tends to respond to successful treatment for active bowel disease. A flare of arthritis might actually be a pretty good indicator that the bowel disease is beginning to reactivate, even though recognizable bowel symptoms may not have appeared. On the other hand, if you had the ankylosing spondylitis–like arthritis with your Crohn's disease, the activity of the arthritis would not necessarily parallel that of the bowel disease, and the arthritis would need to be treated as a separate condition."

"Thank heaven we don't have that situation, at least," sighed Edgar. "Is there any research going on in Crohn's disease?"

What is the status of Crohn's disease research?

Grateful for the change of subject, the doctor replied, "Oh yes, a lot of research is going on, both as to the basic mechanisms of Crohn's disease as well as the effectiveness of treatment. Since the disease was recognized only just over seventy years ago, it is a relative baby among diseases. There is still plenty we don't know about it, and of course there is controversy about some aspects of it as well.

"Dr. William Sandborn, an expert in the study of inflammatory bowel disease, has pointed out that Dr. Richard Farmer proposed the first classification of Crohn's disease from his study of 615 patients at The Cleveland Clinic in the mid-1970s. This classification was based mainly on the anatomic location of bowel inflammation: small intestine—29 percent, large intestine—27 percent, or both—41 percent, with the last group having the most complications.

"Another classification, proposed by Dr. David Sacher at Mount Sinai Hospital in New York about a decade later, further subdivided 770 surgical patients with Crohn's disease into those with perforating disease—49 percent—and nonperforating disease —51 percent. He reported that about half of the patients operated on for either type of disease went on to have a subsequent operation. More recently, several studies suggested that the most useful classification divides the patients at the time of diagnosis into nonstricturing, that is, no bowel obstruction; nonpenetrating disease —about 80 percent; stricturing nonpenetrating—a very small percentage; and pene- trating disease—about 15 percent. But by the time you follow the patients for ten years, the 80 percent with no complications is down to about 20 percent. What does all this mean?" the doctor said. "Over time, increasing numbers of patients get complications, many of which require a surgical approach. About 40 percent of the patients come to surgery within two years after the diagnosis is made, and this is about half of the patients who ever get surgery."

"That sounds like there is probably an operation in my future," observed Edgar.

"Given today's technology, that's probably true," agreed the doctor. "But new medical treatments are being developed all the time, and there is great hope that the present discouraging results can be improved upon. In any case, you are doing well now, so we may have some time. By the time you need them, there may be some alternatives available that we don't have now. One interesting treatment under investigation now is giving infliximab by mouth. That certainly delivers it to the site of disease, and the early results of such treatment are encouraging."

Course and follow-up

Edgar did quite well over the next few months. He was able to get completely off prednisone, and his arthritis resolved. He continued to take mesalamine and tolerated it well. He had occasional gastrointestinal symptoms, just enough not to forget that he had Crohn's disease, but in reality, it was not entirely clear whether the gas he continued to have from time to time was from the disease or the treatment.

Considering all that had happened, he found it difficult to maintain his former level of formality and aloofness at work, and he began to call some of his closest friends by their first names. This was a big step for him, and Miss Perkins—Twyla—and Felix were much relieved and amused by it. Twyla began to accompany him on his regular follow-up visits to the doctor, and on one such occasion, about a year after the dramatic onset of Edgar's symptoms, the doctor noticed that she was sporting a spectacular diamond ring on her left fourth finger.

"Edgar, you're doing well, and I am most pleased," began the doctor. "And allow me to congratulate you and Twyla on your engagement. I hope that I'll be invited to your wedding. What took you so long?"

"Well, Doctor," said Twyla, "we decided some months ago that we wanted to marry, but we are conventional people. I didn't want to go by my maiden name after marriage, but I had a hard time coming to grips with the fact that thereafter I would be known as Twyla Twickenham. I guess that eventually, though, love conquers all."

Disease at a glance: Enteropathic arthritis

Who gets it?

- More common in women than men

- More common in Caucasians than African Americans

- Family history often positive

- About 120,000 Americans affected (25 percent of those with Crohn's disease, of which arthritis is the most common complication)

Joint involvement

- Tends to be oligoarticular and asymmetrical

- Inflammation may be more periarticular than within the joints themselves, but can be destructive

- Ankylosing spondylitis occurs in some patients

Other features and complications

- Fistula formation

- Intestinal obstruction

- Intestinal perforation

Laboratory features

- Acute phase reactants elevated

- HLA-B27 in patients with spondylitis

- Rheumatoid factor negative

Treatment

- General
    - o Adequate rest
    - o Appropriate exercise
    - o Low-residue diet
    - o Education
- Medications for Crohn's disease
    - o Temporary systemic corticosteroids
    - o Aminosalicylates
    - o Immunosuppressive drugs
    - o TNF-alpha inhibitors
    - o Antibiotics
- Medications for arthritis
    - o Aspirin or other NSAID (if tolerated)
    - o Temporary systemic corticosteroids
    - o Local joint injections
- Surgery if appropriate

Chapter 11
Polymyalgia Rheumatica (PMR)

Onset: A bolt from the blue

Jed was lying in bed on a wintry morning, enjoying the warmth and musing over a conversation that he had overheard the day before at the senior center where, since his retirement a few years earlier, he volunteered to help other older folks with their taxes each year. His friend Caleb had been complaining to Harley and Irvin about his prostate problems. Caleb said, "Every morning, I get up around seven and go into the bathroom to take a leak, but it takes me sometimes up to ten minutes to get it started, and then I trickle and dribble and make a big mess around the commode, and it's hard to get my bladder to empty out." Harley was sympathetic. He said, "I get up around eight and go into the bathroom to take a crap. Sometimes I have to sit there for twenty minutes, and then the stool is hard and too big, and it hurts to get it out. Sometimes it's a little bloody." Irvin said, "Well, I pity you guys. Every morning around seven, I urinate without any trouble, and around eight, I have a nice, pleasant bowel movement. Then at nine, I get up."

Jed was glad he didn't have any of those problems. Elsie was still sleeping, but he decided that it was time for him to get up and get ready for his day at the senior center. He rolled over, but when he sat on the edge of the bed, he knew he was in trouble. Every muscle in his body was sore, and he was stiff as a board. As Jed stood up, his whole pelvis felt as if it were on fire. His hips didn't want to move, and his thighs felt unbearably heavy, but he finally managed to get to the bathroom. Raising his arms to get his pajama top off took tremendous effort and provoked pain throughout the shoulder regions. He got his glasses on and looked himself over in the mirror. Nothing appeared to be amiss; there was no swelling in the shoulders or the knees. But what in the world was going on? He had never felt like this before. He was scared, but he didn't call Elsie.

Jed decided to take a shower to see if that would help. He turned on the water as hot as he could stand it, even though he knew that had bad effects on his dry skin, especially during cold weather. He noticed that his hands were not stiff or sore, and he had no difficulty turning the faucets of the shower. He stood under the steaming stream of water, and he slowly began to loosen up a little. The heat felt good, and some of the soreness seemed to get a little better. But as soon as Jed got out of the shower, the soreness and stiffness returned with a vengeance. It was even hard to shave, because his shoulders were so sore. He took three aspirin.

Jed sat at the breakfast table, but he really didn't feel like making the effort to brew coffee, unload the dishwasher (one of his morning tasks), go out and get the paper, or pour his cereal. Although about a half-hour had gone by since he'd taken the aspirin, he felt no better.

Soon Elsie came bouncing in. She was an attractive, cheerful woman of seventy, a couple of years younger than Jed. They had known each other since college and had been married for nearly forty-five years. Morning was her favorite time, and she looked forward to sharing breakfast, sipping coffee, and lingering over the newspaper with Jed. Immediately she recognized that all was not well with her husband, whom she could read like a book. With some alarm, she asked, "What's wrong, honey? Where's the newspaper? Are you okay?"

"I feel like I've been hit by a truck," said Jed. "Even my hair hurts. I can hardly move."

"Were you feeling okay last night when we went to bed? Did you strain something? You didn't seem to be having any trouble then," she said, recalling the amorous activities of the previous evening.

"I was fine. I woke up with this. Maybe it's a virus or something, but I never felt like this before. I need to go see the doctor and find out what's going on."

Elsie called the doctor's office, and Mrs. Babbitt, the nurse, said to bring Jed in. He limped to the car. He felt exhausted by the time they got to the doctor's office, and the soreness was even worse.

The doctor, a young geriatrician who was new to the community and to the Medicare HMO that Jed and Elsie belonged to, seemed very nice. He questioned Jed about his symptoms. Then he asked whether Jed had experienced any headache or visual symptoms. He examined Jed carefully and thoroughly, paying particular attention to the temple areas of Jed's head. Jed had no soreness in those areas, one of the few parts of his body that didn't hurt.

When the doctor had finished the examination, he sat with Jed and Elsie and said, "Jed, I think you have a relatively common rheumatic condition called polymyalgia rheumatica; we call it PMR for short."

"I've heard of PMS but not PMR," observed Elsie.

"It's kind of surprising, considering how common PMR is, that it's so unfamiliar to most people," said the doctor.

"Well, what is it?" asked Jed.

How did the doctor know the diagnosis?

The doctor felt comfortable treating patients with this disease because, even though he was not a rheumatologist, he knew how to treat it, and he knew that Jed's response to treatment would likely be considered miraculous by the elderly couple. "Jed, PMR is a condition that causes pain and stiffness in the muscles, particularly around the shoulders and hips. It typically begins suddenly, and it mainly affects people past the age of fifty. It generally doesn't affect the joints, and therefore it is really not a form of arthritis in most people, although some folks get knee swelling with it. Also, it generally doesn't cause pain around the hands, wrists, feet, or ankles."

"Bull's-eye so far," said Jed. "What do we do next?"

"I want to confirm the diagnosis with some laboratory tests. In the meantime, I want to start you on a medicine that I think will give you a lot of relief."

"What's that?" asked Jed. "Aspirin sure didn't touch it."

"I want you to start low-dose prednisone. Your response to this drug will also help us confirm the diagnosis."

"Isn't that cortisone?" asked Jed suspiciously. A couple of his buddies at the senior center were taking prednisone. Although they looked normal, they were always talking about how dangerous cortisone was and how they were hooked on it. Come to think of it, he didn't know why they were taking prednisone, and he wondered whether they had what he had, since it seemed so common. He resolved to ask them about it.

"Yes," said the doctor, "prednisone is a synthetic form of cortisone. It has a lot of side effects, and if we need to continue it, we can talk in detail about them. For now, I want you to take the prednisone at this dose until we get the lab results back. If you turn out not to have PMR, we can stop it in a few days with no harm done. But I think you probably do have PMR, and this should give you some fairly rapid relief."

"That sounds good to me," said Jed. Elsie nodded her assent.

The doctor gave them Jed's prescription for prednisone, 15 mg daily, and made an appointment for him to return in a week.

First follow-up visit

Jed waited to start the prednisone until the next day. He thought that a good night's rest might just clear up the whole thing. But he was wrong. If anything, he felt worse the next morning, and as soon as he got up, he took the prednisone. By noon, he felt somewhat better, and by the next morning, he felt completely normal. He kept taking the prednisone daily, and by the time he returned to the doctor's office a week later, he felt as though he had never been sick a day in his life.

"How are things going, Jed?" asked the doctor.

"It was like a miracle," enthused Jed, and Elsie had to agree. "All the pain and stiffness went away the first day. I feel like a new man."

The doctor then told Jed that the tests for rheumatoid arthritis, lupus, and other conditions had all been negative, but the red-cell sedimentation rate was markedly elevated to 120 millimeters per hour. "That is characteristic of PMR," said the doctor, "and the rapid, complete response to low-dose prednisone is also very typical."

Jed said he had talked to his friends Frank and Abe at the senior center, and both of them were taking prednisone for PMR. "When I asked them why they hadn't told me what they had, Frank said that he didn't know the abbreviation and couldn't pronounce the name of the disease, but he liked the name PMR, and he would use that to tell people who wanted to know what was the matter with him.

"So, Doc, what is PMR?"

Jed's Questions

What is PMR, and what causes it?

"Well, you know how PMR feels better than I do," said the young geriatrician. "The typical features of it are pain and stiffness in the proximal muscles—the muscles of the shoulders and pelvic region. It often, but not always, starts suddenly, just as it did in your case.

"PMR was recognized as a disease in England before it was recognized here in the United States, and as diseases go, it was rather recently described. Dr. William Bruce first called it senile rheumatic gout in 1888, but it is obviously not gout. Other names for the condition included rhizomelic pseudoarthrosis, humeroscapular periarthrosis, and anarthritic rheumatoid syndrome. It was not until 1957 that the name *polymyalgia rheumatica* was given to it by Dr. H. Stuart Barber. Unfortunately, like many of the rheumatic diseases, the cause is unknown. The leading candidates for causation are infection or autoimmunity, but there is not really much evidence for either one. Some years ago, there was interest in the theory that an infectious agent carried by birds might be the cause because many people who got PMR had pet birds in their houses. Although this was never disproved, it wasn't proven either, and this idea, though interesting, is not accepted by most authorities. Recent wisdom is that the pain of PMR is caused by synovitis, which is inflammation of joint membranes, or by bursitis, which is inflammation of the fluid sacs, or bursas, that cushion and protect muscles from rubbing underlying tissues or bones."

"We have a canary," said Elsie. "Should we get rid of him?"

"No need for that," the doctor said, "because we can treat this disease anyway, and there's no proof your canary has anything to do with it."

"I'm glad of that, because I like the little fella," said Elsie.

"There is also a genetic component to PMR," said the doctor. "It is associated with one of the genetically determined transplantation antigens, called HLA-DR4. The gene for this antigen is also found in many patients with rheumatoid-factor positive rheumatoid arthritis. The HLA-DR4 gene seems to be one of the determinants of autoimmunity."

"Anyway," said Jed, having heard all that he wanted to hear about that, "I seem to be cured. When can I stop the prednisone?"

How long do I have to take prednisone?

"Experience has shown us that you will probably need to take prednisone for at least two years, and perhaps for as long as ten years. Although it is likely that we can reduce the dose almost immediately to between 5 and 7.5 milligrams of prednisone daily, to go below that in the first two years almost invariably causes a relapse. After that, we can try reducing the dose every six months, as long as there is no recurrence of symptoms. Eventually, you should be able to stop the prednisone altogether, although there are some people who need to take it indefinitely."

Jed asked, "Are there any complications of PMR?"

What are the complications of PMR?

The doctor responded, "PMR has a relationship with a much more serious condition called giant cell arteritis, or GCA. This is an inflammation of the arterial wall that primarily affects the cranial arteries, including the temporal arteries, which are located just under the skin in front of the upper part of the ears. If you put your finger there lightly, you can feel your temporal artery pulse." Jed and Elsie both confirmed this as the doctor continued, "GCA occurs in a small percentage of people with PMR. It is painful and causes headache and tenderness in the temporal regions. But the greatest importance of GCA is that it can cause sudden loss of vision that does not reverse.

That's why I asked you about headache and visual disturbances and felt your temporal arteries when I first examined you."

"What if I had GCA?" asked Jed.

"That is a medical emergency," said the doctor. "If you had any signs of GCA, which you didn't, I would have started you on a larger dose of prednisone at the time of your first visit. I would also have ordered a temporal artery biopsy to confirm the diagnosis. People with GCA have a typical microscopic appearance of their arterial walls, the most characteristic feature of which is the presence of large cells with multiple nuclei, called giant cells. High-dose prednisone, started early enough and continued for about six weeks, usually is adequate to prevent blindness from this condition.

"GCA can also cause some other nasty things, such as gangrene of a portion of the scalp or tongue, a strokelike condition, and other symptoms resulting from shutting off the blood supply in the distribution of the affected arteries. It's not a pleasant disease, and I am glad you don't have it."

"Am I out of the woods on that one, or could it still occur?" asked Jed.

"The most common situation where GCA appears late in someone being treated for PMR would be reduction or elimination of prednisone too soon or too suddenly," said the doctor. "We aren't going to do that, right?"

"Not if I can help it," said Elsie.

"You said prednisone has a lot of side effects, Doc. What are they?" asked Jed.

What are the side effects of prednisone?

"Prednisone side effects tend to be dose related and duration related. That means that the higher the dose or the longer you take it, the more likely you are to get side effects," the doctor replied. "You will see the effects of long duration of treatment, but not high dose. Over time, you will see some thinning of the skin, some superficial bruising, and you may have a tendency to gain weight and to lose calcium from the bones, which is called osteoporosis. Some people on long-term prednisone develop cataracts, even when the dose is low.

"Other side effects include hypertension, moon face, abnormal redistribution of body fat to the trunk and away from the extremities, purple stretch marks on the abdomen, susceptibility to infection, and diabetes. These are more common in people on higher doses of prednisone, but they are not unknown even at low doses taken chronically. Some people have psychiatric disturbances induced by prednisone, generally restricted to mood swings but sometimes more severe, and overt psychoses brought on by prednisone are not unknown."

"Man, is there anything it doesn't cause?" asked Jed. "Sounds like it could be worse than the disease."

"The fortunate thing," said the doctor, "is that most of these conditions are rare, and they are also mostly reversible upon discontinuing the drug. They don't necessarily reverse rapidly, however."

"Is there any alternative to prednisone?" asked Jed.

Are there alternatives to prednisone in treating PMR?

"None that works very well," said the doctor. "There were high hopes a number of years ago, particularly in England, that the nonsteroidal anti-inflammatory drugs, or NSAIDs, might work, but they didn't. Furthermore, they provided no protection against GCA. There has been experimentation with drugs that might allow minimization of the dose of prednisone, like methotrexate, but results have been disappointing.

"However, not to worry," said the doctor. "You are doing fine on prednisone, and we are going to reduce the dose to 10 milligrams daily, as of tomorrow. Give me a call in a couple of days to let me know how you are getting along. I'll see you again in two weeks, and we can continue our prednisone reduction plan. Meanwhile, be sure to let me know if you develop any visual symptoms or headaches."

Course

Jed continued his prednisone, and within a month, he was able to get the dose down to 5 mg per day. He continued to feel well. His doctor put him on supplemental calcium and vitamin D to ward off osteoporosis and checked him frequently for diabetes and hypertension. It took several tries over the next five years, but Jed was finally able to get himself totally off prednisone without relapsing. His vision remained intact, and he, Elsie, and Richard, their canary, lived happily ever after.

Disease at a glance: Polymyalgia rheumatica

Who gets it?

- Onset generally after age fifty
- Women affected more commonly than men
- Typically sudden onset

Joint involvement

- Predominantly affects muscle (typically the proximal musculature)
- Synovitis in knees sometimes demonstrable

Other features and complications

- Giant cell (temporal) arteritis may be associated

Laboratory features

- Very high sedimentation rate
- Rheumatoid factor negative

Treatment

- Education
- Prednisone

Chapter 12
Fibromyalgia

Onset: That searing feeling

Mabel was seated—it felt more like rooted—in her accustomed position in her office in front of the computer, scrolling through spreadsheet after spreadsheet of numbers in small print. Her boss, Mr. Fogarty, was the company's dour chief financial officer. It seemed to her that he believed everybody in the company to be an irresponsible spendthrift. In response to his assignment, she was figuring out the next year's budget for her department and trying, as she had each year for the previous five years, to squeeze out another fraction of a percent of cost savings. She was long past the point of shaving off the fat, had probed deep into the muscle, and was beginning in a few instances to scrape against bone in her quest for cost improvements. She dreaded explaining these necessities to her co-workers.

It was already 8:30 p.m., and Mabel was getting bleary-eyed after twelve solid hours of work. It didn't help that she had broken her computer glasses and was working with her bifocals on. This made it necessary for her to tilt her head back to see the screen clearly. Her neck was sore, and when she stretched, she noticed that her shoulders were sore as well. Her upper back was burning with pain, especially around the shoulder blades. Her head ached. She felt miserable, not unlike the way she had felt the last couple of weeks at the end of each day. She looked forward to getting home, sipping a glass of wine, luxuriating in a warm bath, and hitting the sack early. She would feel better tomorrow.

When Mabel got home, the wine hit the spot, and the bath was very nice. During the night, however, she was unable to find a comfortable position. She tossed and turned. She tried lying on one side, then the other, with and without a pillow. She took three aspirins. She tried rubbing her neck. She tried putting heat (a heating pad she had inherited from her mother) and cold (a plastic bag full of ice cubes; it felt lumpy) on her neck, to no avail. Finally, around three in the morning, she got up and turned on the TV, figuring that pure boredom would put her to sleep. At that hour, cable seemed to be showing nothing but movies of unclothed, mammarily enhanced, tattooed young women cavorting about in simulated intercourse with bored-looking, flaccid, forty-five-year-old men, also tattooed. While this held little interest for Mabel, it also did not put her to sleep. And she continued to hurt.

Despite her discomfort, she did manage to doze off a few times, and, as it happens, she was snoozing on the sofa in front of the TV, at that time showing a masterpiece called *Gladiator Eroticus,* when her alarm began chirping at 6:00 a.m. As Mabel struggled to regain consciousness, she became aware that her pain was much worse than the night before. This had never happened to her. Normally, a night of rest would ease the pain. Then she recalled that she had not gotten much rest that night. No wonder she felt so bad. She decided to stay home from work that day to see whether she would improve with some rest.

That night Mabel was even worse. She really didn't sleep at all. The next day, she had pain in all the previous locations, but in addition, her knees were aching, and she was sore around the brim of the pelvis. She was thirty-four years old, but she felt as if she were ninety-four, and she didn't like it. She swallowed a few more aspirins and called her internist.

"Doctor, I think I'm having an attack of arthritis. My mom had it, and she was always complaining about pain all over her body. That's what I have, and I want to get rid of it," Mabel said.

The doctor recommended that she come in for an examination that afternoon, and Mabel was all for it.

Initial examination: What did the doctor say?

After Mabel recounted the story of the last few days, the doctor asked her many questions about her joints and muscles. Were the joints swollen? Were they stiff? Could she move them through the full range of motion? Were the muscles weak? Did they look swollen or shrunken? Were they tender to the touch? Had any of these symptoms ever occurred before? Was she taking any new medications? Mabel had to admit that similar symptoms had occurred before, but that they had never lasted this long or been this severe. The doctor asked about her sleep habits and about her exercise activities. Mabel acknowledged that she sometimes had trouble getting to sleep, especially the last few nights, and that she lived a fairly sedentary lifestyle. She was always tired, and she had become somewhat stout.

"Okay, Mabel, let's get you undressed so I can examine you," the doctor said.

After undressing and donning a small gown, open at the back, Mabel sat on the end of the examining table and waited for the doctor's return. By the time he and Gertrude, the nurse, entered the room, Mabel was shivering from the cold, and her upper body felt as if she were clamped in the medieval torture device known as an iron maiden.

Mabel complained, "You ought to turn on the heat if you're going to leave naked people sitting here for hours at a time."

"Sorry, Mabel," apologized the doctor. "We'll try to get through this quickly so you can get bundled up again."

The doctor then placed his hands on Mabel's shoulders from behind and began probing along the top of the shoulders with one finger, looking for tender spots. He soon found one, and Mabel exclaimed, "Yikes! Do you have to do that?" She was about to complain some more, when he found another spot along the inner margin of the left shoulder blade, producing a bolt of pain that rendered her temporarily speechless, but she soon regained her composure and continued rattling off a fusillade of complaints.

After the doctor finished examining her, having found another dozen or so tender points, Mabel whined, "Well, I was feeling pretty good until I came here, but now I can hardly move. That was about the worst experience I've had this week. I can't remember an examination here that was so uncomforta—"

"Take it easy, Mabel," said Gertrude, interrupting the tirade. "You look like about the healthiest person who's been in this office today. Give the doctor a chance to get a word in edgewise, and I think he's gonna tell you what's wrong with you."

Smiling, the doctor, who had always had a soft spot in his heart for Mabel despite her crotchety behavior, began, "Mabel, I'm sorry you had to go through that. I know it was uncomfortable, but I needed to check you over well enough to find out what the problem is. Actually, the news is pretty good: I think you have fibromyalgia."

How did the doctor know the diagnosis?

"You didn't even do any tests. You can't be certain what I have—I know that. Doctors always do tests. Do some tests, and then tell me what I have," said Mabel.

"I am going to do some tests," said the doctor, "but they are mainly to rule out some low-probability conditions that mimic fibromyalgia."

"What makes you think so?" asked Mabel dubiously.

The doctor began, "Fibromyalgia is a painful condition affecting muscles, rather than joints. So, technically, it's not a form of arthritis. It's a clinical diagnosis based on the history and physical findings, which researchers have grouped into a set of diagnostic criteria. Blood tests are all normal in fibromyalgia, and X-rays show very little as well.

"One of the main characteristics of fibromyalgia is the presence of tender points at some or all of eighteen specific locations. These locations are at:

- the back of the neck—two points

- the sides of the neck—two points

- the top of the shoulders—two points

- the front of the shoulders—two points

- the inner borders of the shoulder blades—two points

- outer sides of elbows—two points

- the brim of the pelvis—two points

- the sides of the hips—two points

- the inner margins of the knees—two points

"If at least eleven of these points are tender, that together with a history of widespread pain fulfills the 1990 criteria for the diagnosis of fibromyalgia. In your case, Mabel, all eighteen points are tender. Other suggestive symptoms are sleep disturbance, fatigue, anxiety, and headache, all of which you have noted.

"So, I don't think there is much doubt about the diagnosis," concluded the doctor.

"All I know is that it sure does hurt. So, why is it good news that I have fibromyalgia?"

Mabel's Questions

What harm can fibromyalgia do to me? Is it crippling?

"I guess it's not really correct to say it's good news that you have fibromyalgia, but it's definitely good news that you don't have something worse," said the doctor. "And almost everything is worse! Fibromyalgia is not crippling. True, it's painful, but it does not damage the painful areas, no matter how painful it is. Think of it like a headache. Headaches are very painful, but in most cases, when they go away, there is no residual from them. Of course, that assumes that they are not due to brain tumors or strokes. And there are many painful conditions—rheumatoid arthritis, for example—that are permanently harmful to the body. But fibromyalgia is not one of them."

"Well, if you like this disease so much, you can have mine. How common is fibromyalgia, anyway?" asked Mabel.

How common is fibromyalgia?

"I don't know of any good statistics," began the doctor, "but it is very common. I have it myself, though not as severely as you do. If we define it strictly, according to the criteria that I mentioned, it is less common but still pretty frequent. And all of us who see patients recognize that there are many patients who don't quite meet the formal criteria, but who have basically the same process going on. In fact, there seems to be a continuum of severity of fibromyalgia that has no exact cut-off point at eleven tender points. Some people with basically the same condition may have only ten tender points. If they don't have fibromyalgia, then what do they have?"

"I don't know, smart guy. You're the doctor. What do they have?" asked Mabel.

"I would contend that they have fibromyalgia because in all other ways they appear to have it," said the doctor.

"Is there anything else that this could be?" asked Mabel.

Are there other causes of fibromyalgia-like symptoms?

"I think you have fibromyalgia," said the doctor, "but there are certain other conditions that sometimes have similar symptoms:

- "One is **hypothyroidism**. Hypothyroidism has a typical symptom profile, which includes fatigue, weight gain, a sensation of coldness, hoarse voice, dry skin, thinning of the hair, and other symptoms, one of which is muscle pain. We can resolve that question with a simple blood test.

- "**Polymyalgia rheumatica** is also characterized by muscle pain, but in addition, it includes stiffness and abnormal blood tests, and it mainly occurs in people above the age of fifty.

- "Sometimes fibromyalgia-like symptoms occur as a **side effect of the statin drugs,** which are used to treat high cholesterol. This seems unlikely in your case, since you aren't taking any of these drugs. These are a few of the more common causes of muscle pain that can resemble fibromyalgia."

"I guess I'm glad I don't have any of those. What causes fibromyalgia?" asked Mabel.

What is the cause of fibromyalgia?

"Strictly speaking, we don't know," said the doctor. "The most popular theory is that muscle tightness causes fibromyalgia, and certainly that seems reasonable, since muscle tightness is clearly a part of the syndrome. If, for whatever reason—for example, sitting for hours in front of a computer—a person's muscles tighten up and remain that way for any length of time, the muscles eventually become fatigued and start to ache. The natural reaction to this is to hold the painful area immobile to reduce the pain. Holding a painful area immobile requires contracting the muscles in the area, but this leads to further local muscle fatigue and pain. It's a vicious cycle of muscle tightness and pain leading to more muscle tightness, pain, and fatigue. The expenditure of energy required to do this results in more generalized fatigue, and this is one of the most common features of fibromyalgia.

"As far as we have been able to determine, however, there is no underlying physical abnormality of the muscle in fibromyalgia, although that is where the pain is. There have been many studies of muscle biopsy material, using the regular microscope, the electron microscope, and nuclear magnetic resonance, without any consistent demonstration of abnormalities. Muscle metabolism appears to be normal, and there is no damage to muscle cells, as there is in polymyositis, an inflammatory condition of muscle in which muscle cells are destroyed.

"There was a famous study done on medical students a couple of decades ago," continued the doctor nostalgically, "in which two groups of students—experimentals and controls—spent several nights in a sleep lab. Those in the experimental group were automatically awakened every time they reached a certain level of sleep called REM—short for rapid eye movement—sleep, which correlates with dreaming. These students developed symptoms of fibromyalgia, while those in the control group, which had not been awakened, did not. This led to the concept that sleep disturbance may play a role in causing fibromyalgia."

"That's interesting. How much were they paid for that little bit of torture? Anyway, how do you know that there is no arthritis? Everyplace that I hurt is at least near a joint," observed Mabel.

How do you know there is no arthritis in fibromyalgia?

"I don't know if the students were paid," the doctor said, "but I do know that there are no consistent joint abnormalities in fibromyalgia, and such abnormalities are required for the diagnosis of arthritis. The joints do not swell, and they are not inflamed. There is no joint damage, even in people who have symptoms of fibro-myalgia for many years.

"The neck is commonly involved in fibromyalgia. X-rays of the neck often show straightening of the normal curvature of the cervical spine, but this appears to be due to excessive tightness of the neck muscles, which regularly occurs in fibromyalgia. The intervertebral joints and disks tend to have a normal appearance.

"People with true arthritis sometimes have fibromyalgia as well, but the fibromyalgic symptoms and the arthritic symptoms are easily distinguished from each other. This is true even when both conditions are actively painful at the same time."

"Wow. All this and arthritis, too? My cup runneth over," Mabel responded sarcastically. "Is there any relationship between fibromyalgia and chronic fatigue syndrome? I sure do feel tired. Maybe I have both."

What is the relationship between fibromyalgia and chronic fatigue syndrome?

"There's not an easy answer to that question," said the doctor. "Fibromyalgia and chronic fatigue syndrome are both clinical conditions of unknown cause, and although there is some overlap of symptoms between the two—for example, both have prominent fatigue—they are not exactly the same. Chronic fatigue syndrome, sometimes abbreviated as CFS, was originally believed to be caused by chronic infection with EB virus, the virus that causes mononucleosis. This relationship, however, did not pan out consistently, and some have postulated that CFS is a form of fibromyalgia in which the fatigue component is more prominent than the pain component. Some physicians don't believe that either condition exists as a specific disease entity and prefer to consider both as merely being out of sorts. Severely out of sorts, you might say."

"I'll say!" agreed Mabel. "So, what are we going to do about this, whatever it is?"

How is fibromyalgia treated?

"Because we really don't know the cause of fibromyalgia and have only some unproven theories about the mechanisms involved, treatment is pretty empirical," began the doctor.

"In my experience, the most beneficial treatment is **a combination of adequate rest and active exercise**—both stretching and strengthening of the muscle groups involved. **Swimming is a very good general exercise** for people with fibromyalgia. You should swim two to three times weekly in a heated pool for at least a half-hour at each session," said the doctor.

"I swim like a rock, Doctor," said Mabel wryly.

"There's no time like the present to learn," observed the doctor. "But if you don't have access to a place to swim, such as the local Y, or if you try it and don't get any benefit, we can go to a more formal physical therapy program. Usually, however, swimming is pretty effective. You have to stay with it, though, and it may take six to twelve weeks to get the full benefit."

"That's just great," Mabel said, oozing sarcasm. "What do I do in the meantime?"

"Since, as I mentioned, we believe that adequate rest is very important, if you are not sleeping well, we can give you **something to help you sleep**. **Temazepam** is a pretty good medication for this, and I will give you a prescription for it, to take one at bedtime. It usually doesn't leave a person groggy the next morning. In the best of all worlds, we should be able to get you off this when the exercise really becomes effective.

"**Muscle-relaxing medications** may also be useful in fibromyalgia, and we have a number of them to select from if we need them. My favorite is **cyclobenzaprine**. It can give fairly rapid relief, but it tends to make some people drowsy, to the point where it can become unsafe to drive while taking this medication. I think we can probably get by without this, but if our other approaches don't work we can consider it."

"I doubt Mr. Fogarty would put up with my taking a nap at work," observed Mabel. "What else do you have?"

"Another medication that is often used for fibromyalgia is **doxepin, an antidepressant**," continued the doctor. "Many physicians believe that depression plays a role in the genesis of fibromyalgia, and certainly people who have the condition for any length of time are prone to become depressed, perhaps another vicious cycle. We may hold off with this one for now because I don't think you are depressed, but we can keep it in reserve in case we need it.

"A lot of other remedies for fibromyalgia have been tried, and that's what often happens in conditions where recommended treatments don't always work. It is probably better to stick to mainline therapies, at least for now, and give them a chance before branching out into the never-never land of unproven treatments."

"What other remedies are we talking about?" asked Mabel.

"If you go to the Web and do a search for *fibromyalgia* or the old term for it, *fibrositis*, you will find all sorts of things, some based on bizarre reasoning, others based on no reasoning. An example is guaifenesin, normally used as an expectorant cough medicine. Most of these remedies are harmless, but there are no data to support their use other than anecdotal testimonials."

"All right, then. Let's do it!" said Mabel.

Response to treatment

Despite her somewhat caustic manner, Mabel liked and respected her doctor, and she resolved to do what he recommended. She immediately had her prescription filled, and she called the local YWCA and signed up for swimming lessons. To her surprise, she actually enjoyed her sessions at the Y and began to look forward to them. She got a new prescription for computer glasses from her optometrist and no longer had to cock her neck into an uncomfortable position in order to see her computer screen at work. And she found that the quality of her sleep was greatly improved with the use of temazepam at bedtime.

Remarkably, there was also a gradual improvement in her pain. It was so slow that she almost didn't notice it. But by the time her next appointment was due, two months later, she was feeling much better, had lost ten pounds, and no longer felt so fatigued.

She recounted all this to the doctor at her next visit. He was glad to hear it and was impressed, among other things, with her leaner appearance. Then Mabel asked, "Are these symptoms going to come back, or am I cured? I feel like a new person. This is the new me!"

The doctor answered, "There's no cure for fibromyalgia, but you've certainly had a good response to treatment. You should continue to keep yourself in good condition with the swimming, and if you do, the symptoms will be less likely to come back. You can probably stop using the temazepam now, but we'll keep it in reserve along with the doxepin and use it again if we need to.

"Fibromyalgia symptoms may recur at times of stress, either emotional or physical. If you continue your regular exercise program, the symptoms shouldn't be as bad. We would, in such circumstances, probably resume the temazepam and perhaps try some cyclobenzaprine along with it. But overall, the most important things you can do are to keep in good physical condition with your exercise program, maintain your weight in its present range, and get adequate rest. That's not bad advice for anyone, whether they have fibromyalgia or not."

Disease at a glance: Fibromyalgia

Who gets it?

- Women more often affected than men
- Very common condition
- Stress makes it worse

Joint involvement

- Painful muscles, generally in the upper back and the posterior neck
- Tender (trigger) points in typical locations
- Joints not involved

Other features and complications

- Headache frequent
- Sleep disturbances
- Irritable bowel is common
- Neck X-ray often shows straightening of normal curvature

Laboratory features

- No consistent lab abnormalities

Treatment

- General
    - o Adequate rest
    - o Appropriate exercise (active rather than passive)
    - o Education
- Medications
    - o Aspirin or other NSAID
    - o Muscle-relaxing medications
    - o Local tender point injections

Appendix A: Participation in Clinical Trials

Should I participate in a clinical trial as an experimental subject?

Participation in a clinical trial is highly worthwhile if the trial is well designed and is looking at an important issue. Such trials are necessary to bring new treatments into general use. Your rheumatologist can help you technically evaluate a particular trial that you might be interested in. You need to realize, however, that the essence of research is finding an answer where none exists, so there is always an element of risk in such trials that goes beyond the risk that exists in everyday medicine. Only you can decide to take that risk, and you can't make a good decision unless you know what risks are thought to exist. Not only is there the risk that the new treatment might not work, but also that it might actually be dangerous in previously unsuspected ways. There are several protections built into well-designed studies that reduce the likelihood of injury to study participants, but injuries do sometimes occur.

Who is in charge?

First, it's important to find out who is in charge of the study and where it's being done. Reputable scientists working at reputable institutions are more likely to perform beneficial, important research safely. Research hospitals have oversight groups called institutional review boards, whose role is to make sure that all the work done under their auspices is ethical and scientifically sound, and that adequate procedures are in place to assure that the patients taking part in experimental treatments understand as well as possible what they are getting into.

What is the study about, and how is it designed?

Second, find out exactly what is being studied and the strategy for studying it. Get the person in charge (the investigator) to sit down with you and explain it, including just how you fit in. Many studies have a controlled, randomized, double-blinded design. In a drug study, "controlled" means that some of the participants are assigned to an experimental group; that is, they get the active drug, and the others are assigned to a control group, who either get an inactive placebo (which can't be distinguished from the active drug by appearance or any other readily discernible characteristic) or get some standard treatment disguised to look like the experimental treatment drug, for comparison purposes.

If this assignment to groups is carried out randomly, it is called randomized. That doesn't mean that every other patient goes to one group or the other, or some such simple assignment scheme. Randomization is a statistically coded procedure that assures that there will be a valid random distribution of study participants to the groups.

If the study is double-blinded, neither the doctors taking care of the patients nor the patients themselves know who is getting the active drug. As noted above, the assignment is coded, and the code isn't broken until the study is completed or there is some other reason to stop the study.

If there is known to be an effective treatment that prevents damage to the afflicted person, as is the case in rheumatoid arthritis, systemic lupus erythematosus, and many other diseases, **it is unethical to deny the most effective known treatment to the control group.** That was the ethical downfall of the Tuskegee study of the natural course of syphilis in untreated African American males. The final portion of that study was done during an era when penicillin was known to be effective against syphilis, yet treatment was still withheld. The conclusion from this is that you can't ethically do a placebo-controlled trial in rheumatoid arthritis, for example, except for a very short-term one.

Is there a safety committee?

Third, look into the administrative framework of the study. Is it being conducted at a single institution or at multiple institutions (multicenter)? Is there a safety committee of disinterested parties whose job is to break the code periodically to determine whether there is a safety issue that may require early termination of the study (e.g., a high incidence of some apparent side effect in the experimental group or a definitively better outcome in the experimentals than in the controls, providing an early answer to the experimental question)? A functional safety committee would have stopped the Tuskegee study. Especially in multicenter trials, no one center may have enough information to recognize that a trial should be stopped early.

Who is funding the study?

Fourth, find out who is funding the study and what their interest in the outcome may be. Sources of funding could include the National Institutes of Health, a private foundation, or a pharmaceutical or device-manufacturing company. Will the results be published even if they are negative?

What's in the consent form?

Fifth, pay close attention to what's in the consent form. Normal procedure is that someone connected with the study should sit with you to go through the consent form point by point, allowing all the time you need to get all your questions answered. In particular, you should make sure that you understand what happens if you have a side effect that causes additional medical expenses. Who pays them? The consent form should also contain a clear statement that you can remove yourself from the study at any time without jeopardizing your ability to continue to receive normal care for your arthritis. Some studies also have a "crossover" provision. This provision enables controls to receive the active medication (at no charge for a specified time) at the end of the study period, if they so desire. When you understand all this, you can sign (or decline to sign) the form, giving your informed consent.

It is very important for the advancement of science and patient care that many fully informed people are willing to volunteer to be experimental subjects in clinical trials. Everyone owes these participants a vote of gratitude for their sacrifice. But no one can be forced to participate, and it is unethical and morally indefensible for anyone to be experimented on without his or her knowledge or consent.

Appendix B: Drug Equivalency Table (Currently Available Drugs)

Generic Name	Brand Name(s)	
acetaminophen [uh-SET-uh-MIHN-uh-fuhn]	Tylenol	FeverAll
ACTH [AY-SEE-TEE-AITCH]	H.P. Acthar Gel	
adalimumab [aah-duh-LIM-you-mab]	Humira	
allopurinol [al-lo-PURE-uhn-all]	Aloprim	Zyloprim
anakinra [aah-nuh-KIN-ruh]	Kineret	
auranofin [or-AN-uh-fin] (oral gold)	Ridaura	
azathioprine [ay-zuh-THIGH-uh-prin]	Imuran	Azasan
celecoxib [SEL-uh-cox-ib]	Celebrex	
chondroitin sulfate [kon-DROYT-'n SUHL-fate]	Chondroitin sulfate	
ciprofloxacin [sip-roh-FLOCKS-uh-suhn]	Cipro	Ciloxan
colchicine [KOHL-tschuh-seen]	Colchicine	
cyclobenzaprine [sigh-klo-BEN-zuh-preen]	Flexeril	
cyclophosphamide [sigh-klo-FAHS-fuh-mide]	Cytoxan	Neosar
diclofenac [dye-KLO-fen-ak]	Arthrotec	Voltaren
	Cataflam	Solaraze
diflunisal [dye-FLOON-uh-sall]	Dolobid	
doxepin [DOCK-suh-puhn]	Sinequan	Zonalon
d-penicillamine [DEE-pen-uh-SILL-uh-meen]	Cuprimine	Depen
etanercept [ee-TAN-ur-sept]	Enbrel	
ethambutol [eh-THAHM-byou-tohl]	Myambutol	
etodolac [EE-toh-DOH-lak]	Lodine	
fenoprofen [FEN-o-pro-fuhn]	Nalfon	

flurbiprofen [FLOOR-be-pro-fuhn]	Ansaid	Ocufen
folic acid [FOH-lik ASS-uhd]	Sold under the generic name	
glucosamine [glew-KOH-suh-meen]	Glucosamine	
hydroxychloroquine [hi-DROCKS-ee-KLOR-uh-kwin]	Plaquenil	
hylan G-F 20 [HIGH-luhn] (also known as hyaluronate sodium derivative)	Synvisc	
ibuprofen [eye-byou-PRO-fen]	Advil	Reprexain
	Nuprin	Vicoprofen
	Motrin	
indomethacin [in-dough-METH-uh-sin]	Indocin	
infliximab [in-FLIKS-uh-mab]	Remicade	
isoniazid [eye-soh-NYE-uh-zid]	Nydrazid	Isoniazid (frequently called INH)
ketoprofen [KEE-toh-pro-fuhn]	Oruvail (old name: Orudis)	
leflunomide [luh-FLEW-nuh-muhd]	Arava	
loperamide [lo-PEAR-uh-mide]	Imodium	
meclofenamate [MEK-loh-FEN-uh-mate]	Meclofenamate (old name: Meclomen)	
meloxicam [mehl-OCKS-uh-kam]	Mobic	
mesalamine [meh-SAHL-uh-meen]	Asacol	Canasa
	Pentasa	Rowasa
mesna [MESS-nuh]	Mesnex	
methotrexate [meth-oh-TRECKS-eight]	Rheumatrex	
metronidazole [MEH-troh-NIDE-uh-zohl]	Flagyl	Noritate
nabumetone [na-BYOU-muh-tone]	Relafen	
naproxen [na-PROCK-sen]	Naprosyn	Anaprox
	Aleve	Naprelan

omeprazole [oh-MEP-ruh-zohl]	Prilosec	Zegerid
ondansetron [awn-DANCE-uh-trawn]	Zofran	
piroxicam [peer-OCKS-ee-kam]	Feldene	
prednisone [PRED-nuh-sone]	Deltasone	
probenecid [pro-BEN-uh-sid]	Probenecid (old name: Benamid)	
pyrazinamide [peer-uh-ZIN-uh-mid]	Pyrazinamide	
rifampin [ruh-FAM-puhn]	Rifadin	
salsalate [SAL-suh-late]	Disalcid	Salflex
sulfasalazine [suhl-fuh-SAL-uh-zeen]	Azulfidine	
sulindac [SUHL-uhn-dak]	Clinoril	
temazepam [teh-MAZ-uh-pam]	Restoril	
tolmetin [TOL-meh-tuhn]	Tolectin	
warfarin [WAR-fuh-rin]	Coumadin	

Appendix C: Glossary

acute phase reactants (APR)   Common, nonspecific blood tests for inflammation. Sedimentation rate and C-reactive protein (CRP) level are the most frequently used. When elevated, the interpretation is that there is inflammation somewhere in the body.

AIDS   Acronym for acquired immunodeficiency syndrome, a disease caused by the human immunodeficiency virus (HIV). This virus destroys certain blood cells that play an important role in immunity (T-helper cells), leading to reduced ability to resist certain types of infection.

amyloidosis   Disease caused by deposition of protein-containing material in numerous organs (e.g., kidneys, liver, heart, etc.), impairing their ability to function. Amyloidosis typically occurs in people with long-standing inflammatory diseases, such as rheumatoid arthritis or tuberculosis.

antibodies   Circulating proteins produced by lymphocytes, which are elicited by and bind specifically to foreign proteins or polysaccharides called antigens, leading to destruction or clearance of the latter from the body. Antibodies are one of the body's main specific (immune) defenses against infection. Immunization leads to production of specific antibodies.

antimalarial drugs   A class of drugs effective against the organisms that cause malaria. These drugs are used to treat or prevent malaria. An example is hydroxychloroquine.

antimetabolic drugs	A class of drugs that inhibit cellular replication and reproduction. Often used to treat cancers or to suppress the immune system. An example is methotrexate.
aplastic anemia	Reduced levels of red blood cells caused by very low blood-cell production in the bone marrow. May be accompanied by low white blood-cell and platelet counts, a condition known as pancytopenia.
arthralgia	Pain in joints.
arthritis	Inflammation in joints.
aseptic necrosis	Localized bone death, usually near a joint (especially the hip, shoulder, or knee), often caused by high-dose corticosteroid treatment. Also called avascular necrosis.
autoantibody	An antibody (see **antibodies**) against components of one's own body. Examples include rheumatoid factor, antinuclear antibody, anticardiolipin, and many others.
autoimmunity	A condition in which the immune system inappropriately attacks one's own tissues and organs, thereby causing disease, either through autoantibodies (see **autoantibody**) or other immune modalities.
avascular necrosis	Localized bone death, usually near a joint (especially the hip, shoulder, or knee), often caused by high-dose corticosteroid treatment. Also called aseptic necrosis.
bamboo spine	Fused spine in advanced ankylosing spondylitis, with a typical X-ray appearance that resembles a bamboo branch.

birefringence	Polarized light transmission property of certain crystals in which the light beam is rotated to make the crystals visible against a black field produced by viewing microscopically through crossed polarizing filters (polarized light microscopy). Aids identification of uric acid crystals (gout) and calcium pyrophosphate dihydrate (CPPD) crystals (pseudogout) in synovial fluid.
bone marrow	Tissue in the center of many bones where blood cells are manufactured.
bone spurs	Overgrowth (hypertrophy) of bone at sites of irritation, typically seen in osteoarthritis.
Bouchard's nodes	Bony protuberances at the proximal interphalangeal (PIP) joints, often seen in osteoarthritis of the hands. See **proximal interphalangeal (PIP) joints**. Named for Charles-Joseph Bouchard (1837–1915), a French pathologist who described this phenomenon.
bursitis	Inflammation in a sac of synovial fluid outside a major joint that normally cushions the rubbing interface between large muscles and bones produced by movement of the joint. Most common at the shoulder, hip (trochanteric bursitis), and the medial aspect of the knee (anserine bursitis).
carpal tunnel syndrome	Numbness, often accompanied by pain, in the thumb, index finger, and long finger, due to pressure on the median nerve at the wrist. Frequently occurs in rheumatoid arthritis, but can be seen in many other conditions as well.
cartilage	Fibrous tissue, commonly called gristle, that acts as a shock absorber in joints. Formed from a protein (collagen), glucosamine, and chondroitin sulfate.

chemotherapy	Treatment with drugs that kill or arrest the reproduction of cells. Normally used to treat cancer, but also used in autoimmune (see **autoimmunity**) diseases to suppress the immune system.
chondroitin sulfate	One of the components of connective tissue, especially bone and cartilage. See **glucosamine**.
chronic fatigue syndrome	A condition of unknown cause characterized by extreme fatigue for more than six months, often accompanied by impairment in short-term memory or concentration; sore throat; tender lymph nodes; muscle pain; multijoint pain without swelling or redness; headaches of a new type, pattern, or severity; unrefreshing sleep; and postexertional malaise lasting more than twenty-four hours.
complication	An unexpected, adverse effect of a disease or treatment. Amyloidosis and carpal tunnel syndrome are complications of rheumatoid arthritis. Aseptic necrosis is a complication of corticosteroid treatment.
corticosteroid	A class of drugs structurally resembling and mimicking the effects of hydrocortisone, the principal hormone produced by the adrenal cortex. The most commonly used corticosteroid is prednisone.
C-reactive protein (CRP)	A protein produced by the liver and released into the bloodstream when there is active, acute inflammation somewhere in the body, for example, in the joints of people with arthritis.
culture	A laboratory test for infection that consists of growing and identifying a germ (bacterium, fungus, or virus) from a sample of body fluid in an appropriate medium. For example, culturing synovial fluid (see **synovial fluid**) enables us to diagnose infectious arthritis.

cyclooxygenase	An enzyme that enables the formation (synthesis) of inflammatory chemicals called prostaglandins.
cytokines	Chemicals produced by cells in response to a stimulus that act on target cells, resulting in a biological effect. An example is tumor necrosis factor-alpha (TNF-alpha), produced by antigen-stimulated lymphocytes, acting on inflammatory cells, resulting in inflammation.
disease-modifying antirheumatic drug (DMARD)	A class of drugs that, when used to treat rheumatoid arthritis, suppress the disease effectively enough to slow or prevent joint damage. The most widely used example is methotrexate.
distal interphalangeal (DIP) joints	The outermost joints of the fingers.

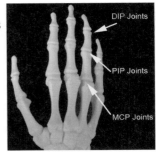

Skeletal model of a hand, showing the locations of distal and proximal interphalangeal joints and metacarpophalangeal joints.

episcleritis	Inflammation of the outermost layer of the white part of the eye, just beneath the clear protective membrane (conjunctiva). Produces a painful, "bloodshot" eye.
erosion	In arthritis, local bone loss at the margin of a joint, as seen on X-ray. Erosions indicate significant damage to cartilage and bone.
fistula	An abnormal channel from a site of inflammation to the skin surface, through which inflammatory fluid can escape. Fistulas, sometimes called fistulous tracts, from the intestine to the skin surface near the anus are common in Crohn's disease.

giant cell arteritis (GCA)	Inflammation in the walls of medium-size arteries, most typically the temporal arteries, sometimes accompanying polymyalgia rheumatica (PMR). So named because of the presence of "giant cells" with multiple nuclei in the areas of inflammation. Carries a high risk of visual loss.
glucosamine	One of the components of connective tissue, especially bone and cartilage. See **chondroitin sulfate**.
gluten	A protein found in wheat products, to which people can become allergic.
Heberden's nodes	Bony protuberances at the distal interphalangeal (DIP) joints, often seen in osteoarthritis of the hands. See **distal interphalangeal (DIP) joints**. Named for English physician William Heberden (1710–1801), who described this phenomenon.
histocompatibility (HLA) antigens	Genetically determined proteins on cell surfaces that act as foreign antigens when organs are transplanted from one individual to another unless there is a match between the two individuals.
HLA-B27	A histocompatibility antigen usually found in people with ankylosing spondylitis, reactive arthritis, and some other seronegative spondyloarthropathies.
immunosuppressive drugs	Pharmaceuticals that suppress immune responsiveness. Often used to treat autoimmune diseases.
inflammation	The body's reaction to many injurious agents. It is generally characterized by accretions of cells attacking the injurious agent and in the process causing swelling, redness, warmth, and tenderness. It is the main process involving the joints in arthritis.

informed consent	A formal agreement, signed by a patient or patient's legal representative, to have a procedure done, to share protected medical information, or to participate in research, acknowledging that the potential risks and benefits have been satisfactorily explained. For participation in clinical trials, informed consent forms must be approved by the institutional review board of the sponsoring institution.
interleukin	A cytokine (see **cytokines**) produced by lymphocytes acting on other lymphocytes and inflammatory cells. Designated by number, i.e., IL-1, IL-2, etc.
iritis	Inflammation of the iris (colored portion) of the eye. This term is often used interchangeably with *uveitis*, or inflammation of the uveal layer of the eye, of which the iris is a part.
Koebner's phenomenon	Formation of an inflamed track along the course of a light scratch on the skin. Named for Heinrich Köbner, a nineteenth-century German dermatologist, who described this phenomenon, which is seen in psoriasis and adult-onset Still's disease.
metabolic syndrome	The combination of central obesity, high blood pressure, insulin resistance, and abnormal blood lipids. Also called metabolic syndrome X.
metacarpophalangeal (MCP) joint	The knuckle joints at the bases of the fingers.
mg	Milligrams
monoarticular	Affecting a single joint. An example of monoarticular arthritis (sometimes called monoarthritis) would be an attack of gout in one joint of the big toe or an infection in one knee.

monoclonal antibody	An antibody (see **antibodies**) produced by a single clone of plasma cells (the cells that produce antibodies). Such antibodies are generally "manufactured" in tissue culture and harvested for use in treatment (e.g., infliximab) or laboratory testing.
myalgia	Muscular pain.
nonsteroidal anti-inflammatory drug (NSAID)	Class of drugs that reduce inflammation by inhibiting an enzyme (cyclooxygenase) responsible for synthesis of inflammatory chemicals called prostaglandins. These drugs are not chemically related to hydrocortisone, thus the term *nonsteroidal*.
oligoarticular	Affecting a small but unspecified number of joints. Synonymous with *pauciarticular*.
ophthalmologist	Physician (MD or DO) specializing in diseases of the eye and their surgical treatment.
optometrist	Practitioner (OD) specializing in nonsurgical treatment of eye problems, generally focused on testing and fitting for glasses or contact lenses.
pauciarticular	Affecting a small but unspecified number of joints. Synonymous with *oligoarticular*.
physiatrist	Physician (MD or DO) specializing in physical medicine (the use of physical treatments for musculoskeletal and neurological problems) and rehabilitation.
physical therapist	Practitioner trained to supervise exercise and the use of modalities such as heat, hydrotherapy, massage, etc., to relieve musculoskeletal problems.
polyarticular	Affecting a large but unspecified number of joints.

prostaglandins	Chemicals derived from 20-carbon fatty acids under the influence of cyclooxygenase enzymes, many of which have inflammatory effects.
proximal interphalangeal (PIP) joints	The innermost joints of the fingers, between the metacarpophalangeal and distal interphalangeal joints.
psoriasis	A common skin disease characterized by a scaling, sometimes itching, red eruption, typically distributed to the scalp, elbows, knees, and areas around the umbilicus (belly button), anus, and ear canals. Often accompanied by damage to the fingernails and toenails.
psychiatrist	A physician (MD or DO) specializing in the diagnosis and treatment of mental and emotional disorders, using the full range of therapeutic modalities, including drugs.
psychologist	A practitioner specializing in the diagnosis and treatment of mental and emotional disorders, using nonmedical therapeutic modalities such as psychotherapy.
recombinant DNA technology	Laboratory methods of manipulating DNA (the chemical structures that contain genes) at the molecular level. These techniques underlie the scientific field of molecular biology.
rheumatism	A nonspecific term that generally refers to aching and pains in joints and muscles.
rheumatoid factor	An autoantibody (see **autoantibody**) that reacts with a normal blood protein called immuno-globulin G (IgG), forming antigen-antibody (immune) complexes. Immunoglobulins are blood proteins that contain all antibody activity. IgG is one of five classes of immunoglobulins (IgM, IgG, IgA, IgD, and IgE) in humans. Rheumatoid factor is found in the blood of 80 percent of individuals with rheumatoid arthritis, but it is also present in many individuals with other conditions, especially chronic infections.

rheumatologist	A physician (MD or DO) specializing in the diagnosis and treatment of rheumatic disorders, including various forms of arthritis and other inflammatory conditions.
sacroiliac joint	The joint between the sacrum (the lowest five vertebrae) and the ilia (largest bones of the pelvis). Anchors the pelvis to the spine.
sarcoidosis	Inflammatory disease of unknown cause resembling tuberculosis. Probably autoimmune in nature.
scleritis	Inflammation of the white layer of the eye (sclera). Can be destructive, especially in rheumatoid arthritis, if not treated.
scleromalacia	Softening and possible perforation of the white layer of the eye (sclera) caused by untreated scleritis.
sedimentation rate	Blood test, the most common form of which is called the Westergren sedimentation rate, that measures the rate at which red blood cells settle in a special tube. Generally expressed in millimeters per hour. Used as a test for inflammation, but can be confounded by a variety of other factors, for example, high blood sugar, anemia, low or high blood proteins.
sign	Evidence of disease that can be observed, e.g., swelling of a joint. Contrasts with symptoms, which are subjective and can be reported only by the patient, e.g., pain in a joint.
Sjögren's syndrome	The combination of dry mouth, dry eyes, and often arthritis. Can occur as a primary condition (i.e., Sjögren's disease) or a manifestation of some other disease (such as rheumatoid arthritis, systemic lupus erythematosus, or scleroderma).

spondyloepiphyseal dysplasia	Hereditary malformation of the vertebrae and extremities, resulting in short stature with short trunk and short limbs. Can lead to early development of osteoarthritis.
symptom	Subjective evidence of disease that cannot be observed, but can be reported only by the patient, e.g., pain in a joint. Contrasts with signs of disease, which can be observed, e.g., swelling of joints.
syndrome	A group of symptoms and/or signs that occur together as a secondary feature of various underlying diseases. An example is carpal tunnel syndrome, which can occur secondary to rheumatoid arthritis, myxedema, amyloidosis, multiple myeloma, repetitive trauma, etc.
synovial fluid	Fluid within a joint.
synovitis	Inflammation of the joint-lining tissue, called the synovium.
temporal arteritis	Inflammation of the temporal arteries, generally characterized by the presence of "giant cells" and often used synonymously with *giant cell arteritis* (GCA). GCA may affect the walls of any large or medium-size arteries, most typically the temporal arteries, sometimes accompanying polymyalgia rheumatica (PMR). See also **giant cell arteritis**.
tender point	Point of muscular tenderness in fibromyalgia at eleven typical locations.
tendinitis	Inflammation of a tendon. Also called tendonitis.
tophus	Aggregation of monosodium urate (MSU) crystals, usually under the skin, resulting in a lump that can be felt and/or seen, in gout.
trigger point	Point of muscular tenderness in fibromyalgia at eleven typical locations. Also called tender point, the preferred term.

tumor necrosis factor-alpha (TNF-alpha)	Cytokine (see **cytokines**) critical to inflammation in many rheumatic diseases, especially rheumatoid arthritis. So called because TNF-alpha is also responsible for breakdown of tumor cells induced by immune response against a tumor.
uveitis	Inflammation of the uveal (pigmented) layer of the eye.
valgus deformity	Generally in reference to the knee: knock-knee deformity in which the axis of the leg is displaced laterally from the axis of the thigh.
vasculitis	Group of diseases characterized by inflammation of the walls of blood vessels. Classified by the size of vessels involved, whether they are arteries or veins, and the nature of the inflammation.
xanthine oxidase	Enzyme responsible for the breakdown of purines from the nuclei of dying cells to uric acid. Can be blocked by allopurinol, used to reduce the concentration of uric acid and urates in blood and joints.

Appendix D: Resources

Books and other sources of the printed word are wonderful, but they have one major drawback: once the last word is written, they begin to go out of date. And few types of information become obsolete faster than medical information. As Thierry Poynard and colleagues told us in a fascinating article entitled "Truth Survival in Clinical Research: An Evidence-Based Requiem?" published in the *Annals of Internal Medicine* in 2002, the half-life of medical truth is about forty-five years, and about half of what we "knew" to be true forty-five years ago, we now "know" to be false! That's why it is so critically important to have sources of information that are continuously updated and corrected.

Fortunately, in the modern era, we have the Internet, a source of information that is capable of being updated as frequently as necessary to keep it current. Although the Internet is a rich resource for current information, it can be a mixed blessing, since not everything on the Internet is equally credible or current. There is no central clearing-house or quality control mechanism for Internet information that assures its currency or correctness. For that reason, a bit of guidance directed at the use of the Internet should be helpful, and I will attempt to provide it here.

If one enters the word "arthritis" into the Google search engine, the result is 12,600,000 "hits" in 0.1 second! Narrowing the topic to "rheumatoid arthritis" reduces the yield to 2,710,000 references. Phenomenal as that is, and while there may be a great deal of useful information buried in such results, unless a person has a lot of time to sift through such a massive data dump, along with the expertise to critically evaluate it, it's not particularly helpful.

Instead, I suggest going to trustworthy sources of information and seeing what they can tell you about the topic of interest. A few such institutional sources include The Cleveland Clinic (www.clevelandclinic.org, then click Departments & Services, and finally Rheumatology and Arthritis); the Mayo Clinic (www.mayoclinic.com, then click Diseases and Conditions, and finally Arthritis under "A"); the Arthritis Foundation (www.arthritis.org, then click Conditions and Treatments at the top of the page, then Disease Center, third from the top at the left side of the page, then search for the disease you are looking for in the alphabetical list); the American College of Rheumatology (www.rheumatology.org, mainly aimed at professionals, limited utility for consumers, but disease classification criteria may be of interest); the Centers for Disease Control and Prevention (www.cdc.gov, then click Diseases and Conditions on the left side of the page, then click Arthritis for general information about arthritis); the National Institute of Arthritis and Musculoskeletal and Skin

Diseases (www.niams.nih.gov, then click Health Information on the left side of the page, then select the disease of interest from the alphabetized list); and the websites of many universities, primarily those with medical schools. The details of looking through these websites may change without notice.

If you are looking for the most up-to-date information on a very narrow topic and don't mind wading through some technical language, you can go directly to the scientific literature via the Medline database, maintained online by the National Library of Medicine. Access to this database is free to the public. It catalogs all articles appearing in the peer-reviewed medical literature throughout the United States and most of the rest of the world. Using PubMed (go to the National Center for Biotechnology Information at www.ncbi.nlm.nih.gov, then click PubMed in the upper left-hand corner of the home page), one can search the Medline database by topic, author, year, journal, or various combinations of these criteria, resulting in a list of references that meet the conditions you set. You may have to go to a library to actually get the articles you find, but the results are often worth it. A somewhat simpler way is to use the recently introduced Google Scholar service (www.scholar.google.com), which not only returns the publications you are looking for, but also gives the number of times each reference has been quoted in the scientific literature. This is a rough indication of the credibility or importance of the source.

There are literally thousands of other websites of varying value purporting to give reliable information about arthritis and related conditions. Beware of those that promote unusual treatments for which the main evidence is found in testimonials. You should check with your physician before trying out anything you read about on such websites. As I mentioned at the beginning of this book, the most directly accessible source of medical information at your disposal is your physician. He or she can help you find the information you are seeking, give you an assessment of its believability and, just as important, determine its applicability to your situation.

Happy hunting!

Index

Cleveland Clinic Press

The Cleveland Clinic Press is a full-line publisher of non-fiction trade books and other media for the medical, health, nutrition, and exercise markets. Our fall-winter list includes the Cleveland Clinic Guides and our new hardcover imprint, Crile Books.

It is the mission of the Press to increase the health literacy of the American public and to dispel myths and misinformation about medicine, health care, and treatment. Our authors include leading authorities from The Cleveland Clinic as well as a diverse list of experts drawn from medical and health institutions whose research and treatment breakthroughs have helped countless people.

Each Cleveland Clinic Guide provides the health-care consumer with the highest quality, practical, useful, reliable, and authoritative information. Every book is reviewed for accuracy and timeliness by the experts of The Cleveland Clinic.

Crile Books focus on serious medical issues that confront society, with stories of medical drama and important biographical studies of the leaders in medical science and health care.

www.clevelandclinicpress.org

The Cleveland Clinic Foundation

The Cleveland Clinic Foundation is one of the largest, not-for-profit multi-specialty group practices in the United States and is recognized as a world leader in the diagnosis and treatment of cardiovascular disease.

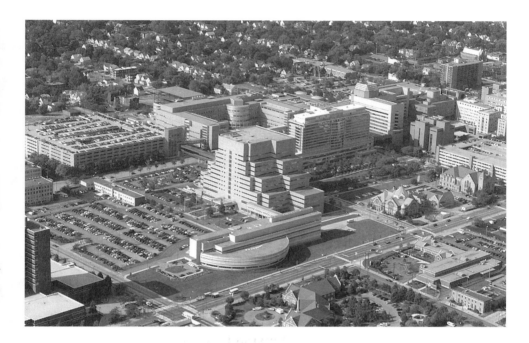

Since 1995, *U.S. News & World Report* has ranked The Cleveland Clinic Heart Center as the "Best" provider of cardiac care in America for 11 consecutive years. In 2002, The Cleveland Clinic Heart Center performed 3,825 cardiac surgical procedures, substantially more than any other center in the U.S. Of those procedures, 520 were minimally invasive valve repairs/replacements with a 0% mortality rate, again representing the largest subspecialty practice in the nation. The Cleveland Clinic Heart Center performed 60 heart transplants in 2002, and its overall mortality rate for all cardiac surgical procedures was 2.0%.

www.ccf.org

HPARW 616
.722
C647

CLOUGH, JOHN D.
ARTHRITIS

PARK PLACE
06/06

Friends of the
Houston Public Library